CONTENTS

FOREWORD

This century began with an industrial revolution that reshaped our society and we are now about to enter the new millennium on the crest of an IT revolution that will have an even more dramatic impact on all our lives.

Information technology (and the Internet in particular) is now routinely enhancing the quality of our day-to-day lives through the access it gives to services and information that we couldn't even have imagined only five years ago. Day-by-day the range of services we can access without leaving our homes increases and the advent of interactive digital TV in the next few years will propel all of us much further and much faster into 'cyberlife'.

Against this background the record of the NHS in exploiting new technology for the benefit of its customers is feeble! To justify this assertion it is a fact that the Americans can get an elderly man to the moon and back (a distance of 250 000 miles), faster than most NHS hospitals can turn round a laboratory investigation for a general practitioner not more than a few miles away.

To be serious (well, actually I am being serious) it really is time that the managerial and professional leaders in the NHS take a good look outside the closed world of the NHS, and learn from other service industries how to exploit new information and communication technologies to improve service quality, speed and availability.

All of us who wrestle in the NHS with the twin pressures of demand and resources need to recognise and adapt to a world where technology offers ways of working that didn't exist only a few years ago. The same creative thinking that has justified email and teleconferencing facilities for managers throughout the NHS should now be applied routinely to the exploitation of IT to support the patient care process.

Ten years from now much of what we regard as futuristic will be in place. The NHS needs to open its collective mind and learn fast!

Frank Burns
Chief Executive, Wirral Hospital NHS Trust
Former Head of NHS IT
October 1999

PREFACE

Why does the NHS get itself into such a mess over IT issues? Computers and all that stuff is easy, isn't it. Kids in their bedrooms are making websites and contacting the world. We even heard about one family who have to email their son from the kitchen to his bedroom, to tell him his dinner is ready!

When the history of the NHS is finally written, it will be littered with stories about NHS IT failures. We'll look back and laugh. The trouble is, it wasn't funny at the time and it wasn't funny for the NHS managers who found IT to be severely career limiting, and it wasn't funny for the suppliers who got so much of it badly wrong and wasted so much time and energy on a customer who didn't really know what it wanted.

The big question for the NHS is, 'what does it want IT and telemedicine to do?' Will telemedicine go the same way as the rest of NHS IT history? We know the Prime Minister is a fan – he saw a telemedicine demonstration and asked, 'why doesn't everyone do this?' Good question. Why indeed? When the bits and pieces for telemedicine have been around for years, why has the NHS never managed to really get to grips with it?

The truth is that the NHS has an unhappy knack of over complicating things and an irresistible desire to reinvent the wheel. Telemedicine is not as complicated as most of the NHS thinks it is. Telemedicine and its derivatives are in daily use all over the world. The NHS does not have to invent anything to make it work. It is all there, out there, somewhere. This book aims to demystify telemedicine, prove that it is not rocket science and help you to implement your own telemedicine projects. More importantly, we recognise that telemedicine is a powerful lever for change – real change, re-engineering change, 'wow' change. Because of that, telemedicine is a team thing, it is inclusive and not the preserve of the 'techies' and whizz kids. It is certainly not about rushing out and buying lots of new kit, although we must admit that is part of the fun.

Roy Lilley
John Navein
October 1999

ABOUT THE AUTHORS

Roy Lilley is a visiting fellow at the Management School, Imperial College London. He is a writer and broadcaster on health and social issues and has published nearly a dozen books on health and health service management and related topics

He now works across the NHS to help with the challenges of modern management and new technologies. He is an enthusiast for radical policies that address the real needs of patients, professionals and the communities they serve.

John Navein is a military general practitioner and has spent many years providing medical care in remote and austere environments. He is an assistant professor in military and emergency medicine at Uniformed Services University of the Health Sciences, Bethesda, Maryland and was the clinical director of the Telemedicine Clinical Advisory and Training Team for the Department of Defence. He is a recognised authority on the clinical application of technology and works around the NHS.

He believes that the time has come for a change and that telemedicine will be the engine for that change.

ACKNOWLEDGEMENTS

Dr Brian Bates, Derby PCG

Lt Eric Threet USN, Europe

Capt Dennis Vidmar USN, Uniformed Services University/Health Services

Dr Lars Engerstom, Fallon, Sweden

DEDICATION

This particular book is especially dedicated to the innovators. Those who know that the pioneers get the arrows, the settlers get the land and the government get the taxes – yet still give it a go

Our day will come!

Come gather 'round people
wherever you roam
And admit that the waters
around you have grown
and accept it that soon
you'll be drenched to the bone –
if your time to you
is worth savin'
then you'd better start swimmin'
or you'll sink like a stone
for the times they are a changin'
Bob Dylan

MAKING THIS BOOK WORK FOR YOU

It is something of an irony that there is a book, any book, on telemedicine. It ought to be on a disk or CD-ROM, or even downloaded from the worldwide web. A book on telemedicine? Must be a joke! Well, this is not any book. It is not a book that is designed to be read – well not from the beginning to the end in the conventional way. We know you're going to flick through the pages, we know there will be things in the book that you know already, we hope there will be stuff here you don't know. So, have a flick through by all means. Use the bits that are interesting and useful for you and forget the bits that aren't. Use the book to crystallise your ideas, use it as a basis for brainstorming and thinking about the issues with colleagues. So, don't feel obliged to sit down and read it from cover to cover in a nice ordered way, because you can't. There is no beginning, middle and end.

Instead, flip through the pages and get a feel for what it has to offer. Not all of it will be of interest to you – skip those bits. Pick out the sections that look like they can help. This is a workbook, so make it work for you. Flip through the pages and make friends with it! Do it now and then come back to this page. By the way, because we are lazy typists, we've substituted 'TMed' for the word 'telemedicine' throughout . . . Make a coffee and have a flip around.

 ## Welcome back!

I hope you have come across things in the book that you know already and, hopefully, some things you've never thought of. Perhaps even some stuff to make you think.

Also . . .

There are a number of **Think Boxes** which are there to get *the juices flowing*, to get you thinking *outside the box* and looking at the issues from a different dimension. Some are deliberately provocative, some just for fun.

Hazard Warnings are there to point out some tricky issues, bear traps for the unwary or those without the wisdom to have bought this book.

The **Tips** are short cuts and quick fixes to get you to the answer faster.

The **Exercises** are there for you to address the issues in the context of where you work and what your task is, regardless of your profession or seniority in the organisation. Use them to develop your own thinking or for brainstorming the issues with colleagues. They will form the skeleton around which you can hang the meat of your project.

These are 'techie' bits. We don't really like you knowing too much of this stuff as you'll grow a propeller out of your head and spend your weekends at Clapham Junction collecting train numbers. These are just enough to impress your friends but not enough to stop them talking to you.

There are a lot of questions and no answers. This is not a 'right' or 'wrong' book – it asks the questions in the context of the issues in the hope that they will help you not to overlook an important topic or duck some of the tricky ones.

This is a non-threatening, environmentally friendly, non-genetically modified, unashamedly irreverently written, fun to play with book that tries to make TMed easy.

Write on the pages, rip bits out, argue with it and throw it at a picture of Bill Gates. Use it as a workbook to prove that not everything in life has to be serious to be good. Well, that's the idea – what do you think?

WHAT'S THIS TELEMEDICINE THING ANYWAY?

Telemedicine is from the Greek and not the American!

'Telcos' meaning distance rather than television. Telemedicine is not just visual based. So, before you start doing anything in the world of telemedicine, tear this page out and stick it on the notice board to remind everyone not to get carried away!

We do telemedicine defined as:

Tele- / *teli* / *comb form* at or to a distance

Medicine / *medsin* / *n* the science or practice of the diagnosis, treatment or prevention of disease

Not

Telemedicine / *telimedsin* / rushing out and buying lots of spanking new bits of kit and making everyone's life as complicated as possible by using technical words and creating a tribe of propeller heads

---

LIST OF

ABBREVIATIONS

ARPA	Advanced Research Projects Agency
CR	Computerised Radiology, aka Teleradiology
EPR	Electronic Patient Record
EPRF	Electronic Patient Report Form (EPR for ambulances)
GP	General Practitioner
HTTP	Hyper Text Transport Protocol
IT	Information Technology
ICT	Information and Communications Technology
IPR	In Progress Review
ISP	Internet Service Provider
KBps	Kilobits per second (measure of bandwidth)
NELM	National Electronic Library for medicine
NHS	National Health Service
PACS	Picture Archiving System
POTS	Plain Old Telephone System
R&D	Research and Development
RTDT	Real Time Data Transfer
S&F	Store and Forward
TA	Terminal Adapter
TCP/IP	Transmission Control Protocols / Internet Protocols
TMed	Telemedicine
TRad	Teleradiology
VTC	Video Teleconferencing
WWW	World Wide Web

Section 1

It's all about change

The recurring theme of this book is the fact that telemedicine is not like go faster stickers on a car or a bolt on 'thingamajig for the whatsitsname'. Telemedicine is about doing things differently – it is not a paste over, make over solution. Now we've got that off our chest, here's a question. Will the NHS be the same in 10 years, or will it have changed?

It's worth remembering that the NHS is the world's largest remaining nationalised industry. They used to say the only organisation bigger than the Health Service was the Red Army (*or was it the Indian railway system? Ed*). Whatever, the NHS employs about 850 000 people directly and probably another 2 000 000 indirectly in service organisations, education, research, technology, equipment and pharmaceutical industries. The budget is around £40 billion and rising. However you measure it, it is big! The fact that there isn't anything around that is anywhere near as big, must tell us something.

It is easy to argue that the NHS is everything that British Airways used to be and British Telecom was. But let's be clear, there is no appetite for the NHS to go down the same route as the airline and the former state-owned telephone company. However, there must be some significance in the fact that the NHS is the last remaining big nationalised industry. If we are to view it as a national asset and want it to be around to look after us all in the years ahead, the question becomes – can it survive as it is?

Survive not in the sense of a national institution or a public service, but survive in its present form. Put another way – is the present model for the NHS sustainable?

Sustainable in the same way that we no longer chop down mahogany trees to make coffee tables and we are learning to treat the environment with a bit more care. Can we go on throwing money at the NHS to sustain it? Few political parties have an ambition to raise taxes and the direct tax taken from individual taxpayers is coming down all the time. A quick glance at the table below soon confirms that.

Who's paying for all this?

Since 1979 there are 1.8 million fewer people paying tax

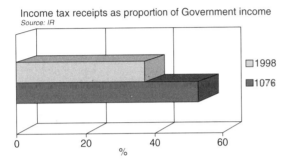

Income tax receipts as proportion of Government income
Source: IR

Governments are learning to be more stealthy when it comes to raking in the taxes. Companies could be hit harder, but they have the ability to set up shop (or headquarters) in countries with kinder tax regimes. So indirect taxes become the only answer. This is a problem too. Despite what you might think is happening in the jobs market, the reality is that most processes are focused on being more productive with fewer people. It used to take 17 workers to make a British Leyland car. Today Nissan do it with just five. However the labour market responds, at best there is an uncertainty about government's long-term ability to raise the taxes we need to run huge public services.

They already have the message and many government departments are doing things very differently. No more differently than what the NHS might regard as its big sister, the Benefits Agency. They got the message a long time ago and embraced technology as a solution to their people-rich systems that dished out benefits and ran up huge operating costs.

They looked to the USA for answers and did a deal with the company that was once owned by the US Presidential hopeful, Ross Perot. His outfit, EDS, pretty well ran the show.

In the meantime the NHS soldiers on in very much the same format it has used since the day it was born. However, internal pressures in health are forcing it in new directions. In the last 10 years or so, average bed stays across all acute specialties have almost halved. They've come down from 10 days to just under six. Bear in mind that this is the average across *all* acute specialties. This pivotal change is a result of two things: the invention of day surgery and the associated benefits of the anaesthetic products that make a certain and speedy recovery possible; and new pharmaceutical solutions to our problems.

If you want an example, think about Roy's Uncle Bill. Bill was a tall, thin, miserable man. He lived on bread and milk and his breath smelt like a drain – he had a stomach ulcer. They took him into hospital, cut his innards open, chopped half his stomach away and sewed him up again. He was still as miserable as sin, still lived on bread and milk – but his breath smelt a bit better. He was in hospital for three weeks and it was touch and go as to whether he would survive.

Roy says that a few years ago, he too had an ulcer and was given a course of pills and never got near a hospital. That's the real change we will see replicated and duplicated in all parts of the NHS. Many of the procedures we take for granted are likely to go the way of Uncle Bill's operation.

Cardiothoracic surgery? With cholesterol-busting drugs, genetic screening and a new wonder drug designed to make the inside of your veins non-stick, who would want to bet their pension that we will still be doing heart by-pass surgery 10 years from now? The sad thing is we are still building huge great hospitals to do it in!

It is the combined pressures of the difficulty in raising taxation to support public services, the increasing consumerism in healthcare, a political difficulty in doing anything about the basic model of the health service and the whirlwind changes technology can bring about, that will all force the NHS to think differently about how it goes about its business.

At the heart of that new thinking is TMed. Think about the top line benefits it can bring:

Exercise

 What are the pressures in your organisation? Compare them with the top line checklist. Which services that you provide could benefit from a re-engineering process based on TMed?

AGREE?

Top line checklist

- More efficient and equal access to medical specialists, less waiting time.

- Reduced patient travel.

- Lower transport costs.

- Fewer and shorter leaves of absence from the workplace (due to rapid diagnosis).

- Reduced number of ambulatory services.

- Lower specialist travel expenses.

- Increased specialist productivity.

- Improved knowledge transfer to primary care doctors and nurses.

- Accreditation of distance learning as part of specialist education.

- Concentration of specialist expertise.

- Reduced requirement for capital infrastructure as services are focused.

- Fulfilment of criteria for service accreditation and clinical governance.

- Fewer referrals to specialists.

- Empower primary care folk to do more with remote supervision or guidance.

- Improved quality of healthcare services due to better co-ordination and continuity of treatment, and better information to the patient.

If you agree with just half of this list you will start to see how TMed fits into the future of healthcare. Indeed, it is difficult to see a future for the health service without TMed being at the heart of it.

Section 2

Nothing is what it seems

D'ya know, there ain't nothing new about all this. Don't let the propeller heads, the anoraks and the gurus tell you anything different. Most important of all, don't let the propeller heads, the anoraks and the gurus take your money by pretending there is anything new about any of this.

Telemedicine is an old idea and most of what we are trying to do today has already been done. Telemedicine – that's the last time we type that word, it's TMed from now on – has been practised since Alexander Graham Bell called up his assistant, Watson, for some help when he wasn't feeling too well. The good old dog and bone (phone to you) has been used to provide medical support for isolated communities around the world ever since.

As far back as the 50s, when men were men, women were women and Freddy Mills lost his light heavyweight boxing title to Joey Maxim (and the world's first kidney transplant took place in the US), the American government started funding various video-based TMed projects. They weren't a great success because the quality was poor and the costs were sky high – but they were trying!

Today it's the other way around. The kit is cheap and the quality superb. It's the NHS that has the problem – the problem of assimilating it all.

There are two places where TMed has been shown to really work well. The first is the military and the second, the prison service.

In step

In the mid-90s, the US military realised it had a problem. They deployed a battalion of troops in the mountains of Macedonia. (In the mid-90s many folk were wondering why the US bothered to deploy a battalion of troops in Macedonia – now we know!) Anyway, they were under pressure to provide a US quality of medical care to the troops whilst they were there. Not easy, particularly as it took 24 hours to evacuate an injured or sick soldier. Plus, the doctor who accompanied the battalion was, as they say in the US, 'just out of the egg'. Translated – inexperienced! The answer was to use a satellite-based, live link, video conferencing system. The junior doctor was hooked straight to the Walter Reed Hospital in Washington DC.

The experiment was a great success and the junior Doc was able to conduct regular clinics with the benefit of an immediate opinion from more senior colleagues back at the ranch. The upshot was that the evacuation rate was cut by 40%, emergencies became 'routine', the junior Doc thought he was Christian Barnard, the commanders thought it was wonderful and the troops thought it was great that Uncle Sam would go to all that trouble just for them.

Lesson: TMed to support primary care works. Yes it does, **BUT** . . . and it is a big but.

Perhaps there is another lesson here. You might wonder why they didn't send a more senior Doc in the first place and avoid the cost and all the paraphernalia of TMed – satellites and all the rest of it.

Well, part of the answer is that it is the tradition in the American military to send the junior doctors forward into the danger zone (the British Army would say they don't have traditions, only habits but that's another story). This goes back to the old days when the troops went 'over the top', including the Docs. The thinking was that you don't want to have your most knowledgeable Docs shot at and 'wasted'. Tradition means that junior Docs still get sent to the front line.

Of course war has changed, at least for now. Ground troops do not often get put into dangerous situations, at least not dangerous in the sense of the Battle of the Somme or Goose Green. These days they get involved in peace keeping, and what they euphemistically call 'operations other than war', around the world at short notice. These days soldiers are highly trained specialists, not cannon fodder and they do need a good experienced Doc to keep them on top form. Priorities have changed, the system hasn't.

So, we can thank the US military for pioneering TMed and we have all learned a valuable TMed lesson as a result. The real solution would have been to change the US military medical doctrine. That would have involved unravelling years of history and habits – so much easier to press the technology button. Lesson? Change what needs to be changed and then think about how technology can help.

In good nick

The benefits for the prison service seem pretty obvious when you think about it. You can't have folk who are banged up in the nick making visits to the local hospital. Well, that's not quite true because they do – chains, handcuffs, prison guards and the full nine yards. But it upsets the feint hearted at the clinics and the prisoners don't like the embarrassment of it all either, unless of course they're planning on doing a runner! More importantly, by all accounts, healthcare in prison is not as good as it could be and TMed is one way to improve things.

A recent Home Office Report suggested that prison healthcare should be provided by the NHS. Seems to make sense but some of the problems are not obvious. For example, a prisoner, referred to a hospital consultant for care, goes on the waiting list like everyone else. But for a variety of reasons prisoners are often shuffled around the prison system from one prison to another and, of course, the average frequency of these moves is somewhat shorter than the average NHS waiting list. This means they're moved before they get to the top and in the great snakes and ladders of prison healthcare they slither to the bottom of the waiting list for the nearest hospital to their new 'home'.

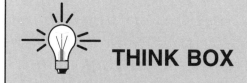 **THINK BOX**

Some estimates reckon that about 35% of inmates suffer some form of mental illness. Mental health remains the responsibility of their 'home' mental health Trust, not the host Trust covering the prison area. Not all need specialist care but many do. So every day British Rail makes a nice little profit from shuffling consultant psychiatrists, social workers and psychiatric nurses around the country for them to visit their patients. Nonsense?

With the greatest respect to the Prison Service it is not the best staffed organisation and does seem to like the odd 'away day' disguised as industrial action. Manning levels are very tight and a bout of 'flu amongst the prison staff can have the same effect. This means that prisoners are unexpectedly banged up and many miss hospital appointments as a result. Who knows how often it happens? And even if they do get there, taking a prisoner to a hospital in itself consumes a lot of manpower and resources which may mean the rest of the prison gets 'locked down'.

As many as one in five prisoners have a serious drug addiction problem. A prison might seem an obvious place to de-tox. Not so. De-tox takes constant monitoring and care which is seldom available in prison at present. By all accounts a steady supply of illegal substances is readily available in prisons and it is not unknown for a 'straight' prisoner to acquire a habit whilst they are in the nick.

From this summary of the problems the prison service faces you don't have to be Einstein to realise that TMed could, and increasingly will, play a part in improving the healthcare of prisoners.

Exercise

List five ways that TMed could improve healthcare for prisoners. (Think outside the jail!)

Section 3

The insertion of technology – sounds painful!

Notwithstanding the fact that TMed has been around a long time, it is only recently that the full potential has been realised. That brings its own problems. If experience in other industries is anything to go by, just inserting technology into a process does not necessarily do the trick. It doesn't always, for example, save real money but it should always increase value for money – there is no point otherwise.

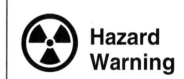

Hazard Warning

If experience in other industries is anything to go by, inserting technology into a process does not necessarily do the trick.

The motor vehicle and banking industries have been there, done that, got the t-shirt and are now reaping the benefits. Do you remember when you used to have to queue up in the bank to get at your cash and you had to be there before 3.30 pm? Now you can go to a hole in the wall at 3.30 in the morning if you want to. Telebanking means you shift your own cash around without ever having to visit the high street and they now even have banks with no branches.

The motor vehicle industry re-engineered its processes based on robotics and IT. In the old days it used to take 17 people to make a British Leyland car – Nissan now do it with five and the car has ABS brakes, windows that go up and down at the touch of a button, air conditioning and receives BBC 2 (at least the new BMW 5 series does), and it all costs the same in real terms as the old metal box of 20 years ago.

If you can stand the man, buy Bill Gates' book *Business @ The Speed of Thought*[1] (his cut goes to charity so that makes it all right). On page 1, he summarises the last two decades from a businessman's perspective:

'If the 80s were about quality [*NHS – clinical governance 1998*], and the 90s were about re-engineering [*NHS is scared stiff to even talk about it*] then the 2000s will be about velocity [*what?*]'.

The medics are well behind.

Never mind the problem, what's the solution?

Change should always occur for a reason. Usually, IT-based change tries to resolve a problem **BUT** . . . yes, there is a big but to all this.

Here's a warning tale:

In the early days of the space race, Russia and the Americans were fighting each other for supremacy and experimentation in space was the battleground. Recording the results of some of the work was a bit tricky though because due to zero gravity the pens wouldn't work. NASA were not the type of folk to let a little problem like that slow them up and so they commissioned space engineers at McDonnell Douglas to design and manufacture a pen that would work in space.

After two years and several million dollars later, they produced a prototype that worked in space, underwater, and upside down. Brilliant!

The Russians bought pencils . . .

So, lesson number one – don't turn to technology for all the answers. Often it is *not* the solution and creates a whole load of other problems along the way. Will your plan pass the 'pencil test'?

[1] Gates B (1999) *Business @ The Speed of Thought*. Penguin, London.

Exercise

Let's turn technology on its head. List some technology-based functions that are over 'technologised' *(Is that really a word? Ed)*. What is there in our lives, that technology has made more difficult? Think of some practical alternatives. Be like the man who invented the wind-up radio!

The key point here is this – introducing technology into a process will require an element (sometimes a big element) of re-engineering of the underlying process to fully realise its potential.

It's like the old joke about the Irishman who was asked the way to Dublin. 'Well', he said, 'I wouldn't start from here'.

Technology is like foundations – best done first. But you have to design your building before you know what foundations you need. And if you're really cool, you'll make some allowance for any developments you might want to make in the future. That sounds sensible but it's not always possible in the

NHS. A situation made more complicated because no one seems to have a long-term vision of what the NHS will look like and what it will do. Indeed, a man from the Ministry told John that visions weren't allowed. 'If you have visions then people criticise them or, even worse, hold you to them – can't have that old boy'. Put 10 gurus in a locked room and ask them what the long-term vision and future is for the NHS, you will end up with 20 answers.

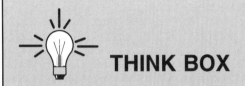

THINK BOX

Did you know it was the Swiss who invented the quartz watch? A bright young Swiss engineer discovered a neat new way to make a watch with phenomenal accuracy using quartz.

He showed his idea to the Swiss watch establishment and guess what? They threw out the idea because the watch didn't have cogs and springs and stuff and therefore as far as they were concerned it wasn't a watch.

Guess what he did? He took his idea all the way to Japan – and you know the rest of the story!

By the way, some of the world's most expensive watches are still made in Switzerland but some of the most accurate are still made in Japan – and they are cheaper, too!

So, waderyerwanna do? Do you want something gold and shiny or something that tells the time?

TIP

It's the outcome that matters, not how you get there.

Section 4

Telemedicine: it's more (and less) than you think

How many times do we need to remind you, telemedicine is not just about television. Go back and have a look at the definition on page xiii. In fact, surveys show that only about one in five TMed consultations involve a television screen – surprising isn't it?

The rest? Cheap, chatty and dead easy to do. How?

Good question, here's a list:

Say what you mean

Time for some definitions

We already know telemedicine is not about screens on the desktop. The TMed gurus define it like this:

> **'The use of information and/or communications technology (ICT) to provide medical care, remotely.'**

. . . might be worth learning this and trotting it out at a TMed meeting – looks like you know something!

By the way, read it again. See, not a mention of a TV, screen, laptop computer, software item, scanner, or any such gismo. Sorry.

Here are some other acronyms and definitions:

POTS. We love this one, it is the best of all! It stands for 'Plain Old Telephone System'. Some say it is at the low end of the spectrum, but don't overlook it. POTS includes advice by telephone or radio (like the flying doctor at Wolumbulla base in the Australian outback).

POTS is traditional, everybody's got one, it's cheap and non-controversial. POTS does the job for up to 40% of teleconsults (jargon speak for telemedicine consultations). Patients ringing up their GP for advice, GPs chatting to the district nurse or a consultant about a patient – they're all POTS. Bet you do it already, so no mystery there.

But you do have to be careful, as it's not the same thing as actually seeing the patient. The GPs know this and have developed safeguards and protocols to protect all concerned when dealing with out-of-hours calls, of which, incidentally, up to 60% can be managed very safely by phone.

And with a little imagination, and learning from the enterprise of others, we can do a lot more. For instance, why do we call patients back to the clinic for review? Why not give them a quick call?

 TIP

Want to talk to colleagues in Birmingham, Manchester, Paris and Southend and don't fancy the travel? How about a BT conference call?

Here's how to do it.

A new service from BT using your normal phone allows you all to talk to each other without travelling. The calls carry a small premium and BT can arrange to have the conference recorded on tape and even arrange a translator service. BT will even give you a separate account with itemised billing so that the costs can be easily identified for the bean counters.

To find out more call BT on 0800 778877 (correct at the time of going to press.

How would a conference call change what you do now? Running a PCG is going to take a lot of talking, talking that's best done on the telephone rather than trying to get everyone together in one place at one time. The nurses may want to discuss a particular issue amongst themselves, chairmen and chief executives may want to chat with the health authority, or a mental health team may want to hold one of those famous case conferences. Do it from your office with a nice cup of tea to hand rather than braving the elements and traffic. (Save time and travel costs.) You can also make rude signs to annoying people on the other end and they won't see you. Silly we know, but it certainly makes you feel better.

Exercise

Make a list of all the meetings you've had in the last three months that could have been held using a conference call. What were the costs in time, petrol and effort? Then think of the meetings you didn't have because it was all too difficult to arrange . . .

Conferencing calling really is what our American cousins so beautifully describe as a 'no brainer'. It's one of those really easy and obvious techno-logy-enabled capabilities that we don't use because we just haven't thought about it. It's cheap, requires no extra kit and the benefits are obvious. So, if you do nothing else after reading this book, make conference calling a part of your routine. Do one now – just to prove you can! You'll feel good all day!

Joint effort

There's a rheumatology team in the north of England who keep in regular contact with their patients by telephone.

They ring 'em up and see how they're getting on. This type of teleconsultation means more regular contact and less aggravation for patients (many of whom are elderly and can't get around very well).

They don't have to go to the trouble of visiting the outpatients department and sit around for hours on end reading out-of-date copies of *Horse and Hound* – at least not so often. Waiting lists start to dissolve before our eyes.

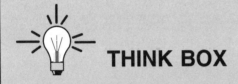

THINK BOX

Perhaps your on call team could be given a stack of notes to go through in the evening, ringing patients up to see how they are getting on, instead of sitting round watching the box. They would probably find it a lot more interesting, unless of course they're advancing their medical education by watching the latest episode of *Casualty*.

GPs likewise can follow up many of their patients this way. The figures vary depending on the specialty but our rheumatology friends tell us they can do about 40% of their business on the phone.

NHS Direct is a POTS system and apparently the biggest telemedicine project in the world, so it deserves its own section. Believe it or not, it started in Milton Keynes. With due apologies to the good citizens of Milton Keynes, can you imagine anything starting in Milton Keynes? Most things seem to stop there.

The Gods of Whitehall are pretty cagey about the number of patients using the system, but it was up around the million mark in September 99 (and not many folk really knew about it then). And it's not that simple – would you want to be on the other end of the phone, at three in the morning, talking to a confused and worried Mum who is trying to sort out the difference between a youngster with 'flu or meningitis?

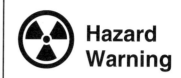

Hazard Warning

Would you want to be on the other end of the phone, at three in the morning, talking to a confused and worried Mum, trying to sort out the difference between a youngster with 'flu or meningitis?

But the fact is, it seems to work. The same approach has been used in the US for years. They started to use it as a way of controlling access to services – in guru speak, 'demand management'. In fact, to date, there have been over 6 million telephone consultations in the US, and guess what? Not one single law suit! In the land where people turn to their lawyers before anyone else, that can't be bad.

How does something with such potential for disaster work? The trick is a clever piece of software that guides the nurse who is on the end of the phone through a series of questions called, in guru speak, 'a decision support programme'.

The nurses take the patient through a series of questions. Depending on the answers, the software guides the nurse to a conclusion and a preliminary diagnosis, together with suggested advice for treatment, referral or follow up. Well, not always a diagnosis but it at least tells the nurse how urgent it is and what needs to be done now (in the middle of the night, so the GP can sleep soundly in his bed).

If you need an ambulance urgently they will arrange one for you; if you need an out-of-hours GP visit, they'll arrange that too. But most of the time they will be using the software to exclude the meningitis and reassure the Mum with some timely advice on what to do. At the moment the scheme is in its infancy but expect to see the system being used for making appointments with GPs, hospitals and maybe even visits from health visitors.

So, next time you feel the need for some health advice, give it a whirl. The number is:

NHS Direct: 0845 4647

Yes, that's the full number – we know it looks short. It's only available in some areas at present but the plan is for national coverage by March 2000 – as long as the millennium bug doesn't get it. Even better, give your local call centre a ring and get them to show you around. If you have any luck send us an email cos' we'd love to know what you think.

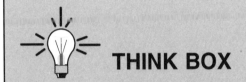 **THINK BOX**

Have you tried calling your local railway station lately? The chances are you won't be able to do so because British Rail (or whatever they call themselves these days) have moved onto a single number across the whole country. So wherever you are you'll have only one number to remember for your enquiries about rail travel (Oh, OK it's 0345 484950). You can also contact them direct via their website:

http://www.railtrack.co.uk/travel/index_personalise.html

Try it, it's easy.

EXERCISE

So, what are the implications for the NHS of a single point of entry with access into hospital and GP booking lists? And bear in mind as you do it that a major London teaching hospital who allowed patients to make their own appointments, registered a reduction in DNA rates from 14% to 3%.

What other areas might a national health helpline move into?

Next funny phrase?

RTDT. This stands for Real Time Data Transmission. 'Real Time' means now; 'Data Transmission' means sending data such as still pictures, X-rays, data from monitors and ECGs down the line.

The expression sometimes includes 'whiteboarding'. You've seen this and probably not realised you knew what it was. Sky TV sports commentators do it all the time. Whiteboarding is when the commentator 'draws' on the screen, usually a line or circle to highlight a section of the picture on the screen. The cricket boys use it to show where 'silly mid-off' is standing; Andy Gray draws over the screen to show which way the United forwards are going to attack. And, the military gurus used the technique to draw all over maps of Kosovo to show what they had just hit.

Some medical applications include the transmission of ECGs from ambulances to an expert either back at ambulance control, the coronary unit or the A&E department. This is important as it allows the diagnosis of a heart attack to be made much earlier, so that appropriate treatment protocols can be embarked upon sooner or even immediately.

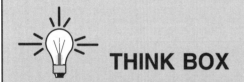 **THINK BOX**

If you're going to have a heart attack, Sweden is a good place to have it. Why? Because in Sweden they use RTDT technology to reduce what is known in the trade as 'call to needle time'.

From the onset of a heart attack, the race is on to inject the patient with some magic stuff and carry out thrombolytic therapy. This works by dissolving the offending blood clot in the heart before it kills off too much heart muscle. The magic brew needs to be injected within 45 minutes of the patient developing chest pain – after that it's all down hill. Every 30 minutes after that knocks a year off the victim's life – figures like that should concentrate the mind.

In Sweden, paramedics are equipped with kits developed by a bright Doc-oriented company called Ortivus. These will transmit an ECG from the ambulance to the hospital. The Doc there confirms the diagnosis and the paramedic administers the magic stuff en route.

Some ambulance Trusts are trying to replicate this in the UK – however, at the moment, thrombolytic therapy is only given on arrival at hospital (or occasionally by GPs in far flung corners of the Realm). Even in urban areas it takes around 40 minutes from 999 to getting the patient through the hospital door – what with inserting the drip, carrying the patient down the stairs, loading into the ambulance and driving through the traffic. That doesn't leave a lot of time, *and* that's even assuming that the call goes out as soon as the patient develops pain – a very big *and*. Some ambulances start to transmit ECGs ahead to the hospital so that the juice hits the vein as soon as the patient crosses the front door. That's a good start but . . .

The interesting thing to consider is the issue of 'pain to needle time'. For the most part in England we're talking 'front door of the A&E to needle time'. In Sweden it's all about '999 to needle time'. What about the concept of 'onset of pain to needle time'?

EXERCISE

What are the implications of the three concepts for the delivery of care, the hospital, the ambulance service and, most importantly, the patient?

1 Door to needle time.

2 Call to needle time.

3 Pain to needle time.

Can we do better?

EXERCISE

What are the barriers in this country to ambulance para-medics giving fibrinolytic therapy en route and do they make sense?

(We'll give you a clue – the right answer isn't yes, although you might get away with a 'sometimes'.)

What would we need to do to bring such a change about?

TIP

This is called 'technology enabled re-engineering'. Good init'? Be sure to show off your new vocabulary at the next meeting and quote liberally from this book! We need the money . . .

More funny words

S&F. Not to be confused with a sexually deviant practice, 'S&F' stands for 'Store and Forward'. This is really just posh email with bits. If you've not come across the expression email, we suggest you try and stop spending so much time polishing your gas lamps and move into the last bit of the 20th century. There's a whole section on email on page 143, so relax!

S&F is different from RTDT because it's not in real time which is good because you can't find a Doc when you want one at the best of times, and S&F means you don't have to get two people at either end of a line at the same time. The consultant can do it over his cornflakes if he wants to. By the way, if a TMed guru who thinks he's really cool starts talking about 'asynchronous TMed', it's the same thing.

Sending email is routine – and increasingly so in the NHS despite the best efforts of NHSNet to thwart us! What you may not know is that it is also possible to attach another file to an email and send it off through the ether. (That's how this book was written. Passed between John and Roy, attached to an email message. It was never printed out until this copy was printed for you!)

The attachment can be a file, a digital photograph or even a CT scan. For example, a district nurse worried about the progress of an elderly lady's leg ulcer may want a second opinion.

So, instead of lifting up the poor old thing and carting her off to hospital, the district nurse can use a simple digital camera to take a picture of the ulcer (and ones of the general appearance of the leg and the patient), up-load it onto a laptop and then whizz it off to a specialist nurse or dermatologist for expert opinion. See, not exactly rocket science, is it? Just like sending a copy of your Xmas snaps to your Auntie Ethel in New Zealand.

OK, let's get serious for a moment. This is inexpensive (cheaper than sending a letter), simple to do (like striking a match) and, used intelligently, as powerful as putting a match to a stick of dynamite placed under the medical establishment.

For instance, we've recently come across an article describing a wonderful new S&F idea being pioneered by that nice

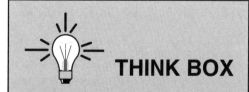

THINK BOX

See, not exactly rocket science, is it? Just like sending a copy of your Xmas snaps to your Auntie Ethel in New Zealand.

Mr Dobson (remember him?). The general idea is that a patient uses a smart asthma monitor that measures their control three or four times a day. At some given point in time, the patient connects the machine direct to the telephone line and through to the consultant, who can assess how good the control is and advise on how treatment may be modified.

What a great idea! No! **Wrong. Wrong, wrong, wrong, wrong!**

What a great use of S&F! **Wrong again!**

This exercise has fallen into the trap that so many TMed inspired solutions find themselves in. Instead of using TMed as a lever for change, in this instance it's being used as an arc welder to reinforce old-fashioned thinking.

Why send the asthma patient's data to a consultant at all? They're busy people and have a lot on their plate already. Even though S&F makes life a lot easier for them and means that they can work from home or the golf course, it still means work. In many cases the digital transmission reverts to a paper printout which takes its place in the consultant's intray.

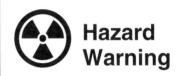

Hazard Warning

Instead of using TMed as a lever for change, in this instance it's being used as an arc welder to reinforce old-fashioned thinking.

How about, instead, sending the data to a specially trained, so called 'asthma nurse'? These highly trained nurses make asthma a specialty, they've received disease specific training, they live, eat and breath asthma and can sometimes be more familiar with issues than the consultant (certainly more than most GPs). And there are more asthma nurses than consultants (and they're cheaper), so it is a reasonable expectation that the service will be faster.

But wait, there's more

Why bother busy doctors and nurses at all? Most GPs would agree that the treatment of asthma patients is, by and large, a giant protocol with a heavy dose of education regarding lifestyle and what-have-you thrown in. That means there's a well-trodden path with recognisable signposts that say, if this happens, go there.

So, what about using the magic new machine to record the patient's condition and progress, and have the machine tell the patient whether or not any adjustment of their therapy is needed? If a new prescription is required or maintenance supplies are needed and control is good, the machine could send a message to the pharmaceutical wholesaler who could post the required drugs, by same day service. It could even measure how much medication has been used in real time and send the order for top up before it runs out. Along the way, a message could be sent to the GP updating him of the patient's progress – GP waiting lists take a further tumble. On the other hand, asthma still kills and if things start to go off the rails, the same machine would pick up deterioration in readings early on and advise early referral before the patient got into real trouble.

If we wanted to be really clever we could programme the machine to bleep to remind a patient to take his/her puffer, warn them when they need a refill or measure their peak flow rates.

We still haven't finished!

Up till now we've only considered the data flow from the patient up the line. What about using the system to send data to the patient. What data? How about things like news of the latest advances in the world of asthma, patient education and seasonal lifestyle advice.

And we're still not finished

The really daring could consider so called 'bundling' of all asthma patients together and have this type of service provided by an outsourced provider that manages the asthma patients to an agreed set of protocols, and is financially penalised for unplanned hospital admissions or failure to meet other quality and treatment outcome targets. PCGs may find this concept very attractive in the years to come.

Now can you see the power that TMed has to bring about system-busting change?

S&F can mean that patients are cared for to a much higher standard. They are no longer subject to the lottery of where they live and who they're seen by.

A fast emerging S&F technology will allow a patient with some chronic disease the convenience of providing a urine sample on sensitised paper which

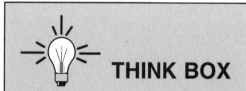

THINK BOX

S&F is a powerful tool that often means that patients can be treated better without having to go to see doctors or nurses or medics, or attend hospitals or clinics. Even geography becomes history.

is then fed into a cigar box-sized machine that analyses the sample (using a process called spectography), digitises the results and sends them off down the telephone line for analysis. This S&F approach is particularly useful for patients on long-term drug therapy such as schizophrenics and diabetics. Clinicians will know whether or not patients are being maintained properly.

EXERCISE

Choose a specialty such as diabetes and design a service for those patients using S&F techniques. Be radical, try and think outside the box and white coats. Don't forget that we used the words 'patient' and 'service' in the same sentence.

EXERCISE

 While you're in the mood for a little S&M – oops sorry S&F – why not have a go at this one?

You've designed your new way of doing business, now look at it and identify the efficiencies that it provides, especially in terms of bricks, mortar and support services. Don't forget that you can do a lot of this stuff from a laptop from wherever you like!

Also bear in mind that an S&F consult takes a lot less time (probably one-fifth of the time, actually) than a traditional one because the provider doesn't have to spend time being nice to the patients and chatting about the latest grandchild before getting down to business. Sorry, brutal but true . . .

'Ask a Doc'

Necessity, as they say, is the mother of invention. The US military knows a thing or two about using technology to solve a problem – 'adapt, improvise and overcome' is the adopted motto of the US Marine Corps. It might just as well be the motto of the gurus who develop TMed solutions for the medical service.

The Yanks had a problem. They have lots of service people and their families spread around the world. Alongside them in these various locations, their primary access to healthcare will often be through a junior doctor or medic. They are pretty good at the day-to-day things but should they need a specialist opinion, who do they go to? You can see the problem. They may be able to get help locally but if they're on a ship in the middle of the sea or serving in a less than friendly environment, they can't pop down the road to the local hospital.

The US military's cunning answer is a service called 'Ask a Doc'.

'Ask a Doc' is based on three simple facts:

- it's easier to move information than it is patients

- a specialist opinion is a specialist opinion and it doesn't really matter who gives it

- geography is history – and when you're in the middle of the Atlantic, nothing is local anyway.

Here's an example of how it works. The captain of a US Navy destroyer under way at sea reports as being sick with earache. The medic flourishes his otoscope (a sexy telescope to look in lug'oles) and sees the beginnings of a nasty abscess in the canal running down to the eardrum. He's not really sure of the diagnosis and he realises that this could be a potentially career limiting situation for him – if he doesn't get it right and get the Captain back to work. Some advice from an ENT specialist would help!

So what does he do? He takes a digital picture of the lesion and emails it with a short history to a central server (with an address along the lines of ent@centralserver.navy.mil).

(*This is obviously not the real address as that's a secret and if we tell you what it is we'd have to shoot you and then you couldn't buy the second edition of this book.*)

It is important to note the first part of the e-address:

ent@

This is the 'generic' part of the address that routes the picture and the history to the duty ENT specialist for the whole Navy. The duty guy may be anywhere in the world – San Diego, Naples or Japan – medical advice never closes.

The message can be forwarded to wherever it is daytime and there is an ENT person on duty or whoever is the least busy.

 TIP

The ENT specialist reviews the material and sends back his advice. He doesn't need to know the patient's rank or name – so there are no issues about patient confidentiality.

Because the data is anonymised, the military does not bother to routinely encrypt medical histories and digital pictures (BMA please note).

Because the data is anonymised, the military does not bother to routinely encrypt medical histories and digital pictures (BMA please note).

The medic on board the ship acts on the 'sound' advice from the specialist and the captain is restored to duty.

 Make yourself a cup of coffee, or perhaps something stronger, and consider the gob smacking, mind blowing, earth shattering, colossal, amazing, major implications that this re-engineering of care delivery, enabled by TMed, has for the NHS.

EXERCISE

 Consider again the three fundamentals of 'Ask a Doc':

- it's easier to move information than it is patients

- a specialist opinion is a specialist opinion and it doesn't really matter who gives it

- geography is history – and when you're in the middle of the Atlantic (or Scotland) nothing is local anyway.

In the blank space below redesign the NHS . . .

Another funny phrase *you must* have heard of!

The Internet

The growth of the Internet has been quite phenomenal and it's getting faster. It's a sign of the times. It took 37 years for radio to reach 500 000 people, 17 years for TV to achieve the same target. The Internet has done it in four years!

It all started in 1969 when the 'way out over the horizon' vision bit of the US Department of Defense – called the Advanced Research Projects Agency (ARPA) – got together with a few academics and industrialists to come up with a new way to send messages. They really wanted to develop their own private network to pass around nuclear secrets without the Russians getting their hands on them (can't be too insecure then). It all went well and the first email message, which included the famous @ sign, was sent in 1972. It developed steadily but it wasn't until 1993, when a chap called Marc Andreeson came up with a way to make web browsing pictorial and easy, that the Web as we know it became a reality.

 Ever wondered what's the difference between the Internet and the worldwide web? Well, the Internet is rather like the road network only built for information. It is a collection of public and private networks that are linked together using a set of protocols called TCP/IP that, if you really want to know, means Transmission Control Protocols/Internet Protocols. The Web is the Internet with pictures. It's that bit of the Internet that exchanges multimedia information, pictures, sound and video (using hypertext transport protocol or 'http').

Our problem with the Web is how to impart just enough words of wisdom without getting too carried away. Put bluntly, the Internet is going to change great chunks of our lives forever. Ask your kids. You can do your banking across it, buy books, cars or whatever else you like. You can use it to have fuzzy VTCs with anyone else who's on it, anywhere in the world, for the price of a local call. You can access huge databases, play the markets or get the latest gossip from your favourite football club. And for a few bob you can even set up your own front window to the World (*see* http://www.roylilley.co.uk). But we are getting ahead of ourselves. We are assuming that you know how to do it. If your partner is a web widow/er already, then skip this bit but if not, here's the lowdown on how to become a fully fledged web surfer.

The basic requirements to surf

You need a computer that has a link to the world. The link can be either down your phone line via a thing called a modem or through the 'network' at work. (The modem converts your computer's digital output into telephone language [analogue].) The computer also needs a piece of software called a 'Web browser', such as Netscape Navigator or Internet Explorer, to enable you to play with http files.

The other piece of the jigsaw (if you're surfing from home) is an ISP or Internet Service Provider, which connects your computer to the Internet. You dial in to their computer which is a part of the 'net and they take care of the rest. There are loads of them and they all give you a slightly different deal. Essentially though there are two types, you can either have one for free (but with the aggravation of loads of adverts) or advert free for about £10 a month. Also, when you're choosing an ISP it's well worth finding out how big their connection to the Internet is because if it's only a couple of bits of copper wire between thousands of clients and the big wide world of the 'net, it will take loads of time for little old you to get anything done. And that will make you very cross, believe us. Ask around your mates to find out what your local ISPs are like.

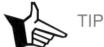

TIP

The worldwide web is worldwide, that's the point, but most users by far are in America. So you'll find it quicker to use when they're all in bed (New York is five hours behind).

A consideration for the jet setters amongst you, is that the really big ISPs like CompuServe and AOL have local access numbers in most countries in the world. This can be very useful because it means that you can easily pick up your email (or your S&F referrals) from wherever it is in the world that you happen to be sunning yourself.

Your ISP will generally give you an email address, often up to five – so each member of the family can have their own. Many will also give you a slot on their server for you to post your own website, if you feel the urge to do that sort of thing.

EXERCISE

What are the pros and cons of allowing Internet access at work?

TIP

Remember that it still costs you local call rates to access the Internet and these can quickly add up over time. So if you try surfing and you like it to the point that you start hearing dark murmurings from your partner or, even worse, if your kids get into the swing of it, sign up your ISP access number with BT as one of your 'families and friends' to get a discount. After all, your partner probably thinks you love your computer more than them anyway, so you're only making the relationship official. Some deals are offering free local calls – but look out for the catch!

Now, just get on the 'net and play. Try Roy's site as a starter for 10.

Log into your ISP and choose a search engine (search engines are awesome things which can search the whole Internet in seconds and find all the sites which are linked to a key word, phrase or address that you put into it). Then type in 'RoyLilley' (one word), press 'enter' and Bingo, you're in.

Get a feel for what it looks like and what aspects of it make it attractive or otherwise (apologies for the photo). Try some of the links and perhaps use the bookshop link to buy extra copies of this book as Christmas presents for all your friends.

But what's it got to do with medicine?

Good question, and the answer is quite a bit now but a huge amount in the future. For instance, one of the best of the search engines is called Yahoo which has a UK version. Type in:

http://www.yahoo.co.uk/Health/Diseases_and_Conditions/

You will end up with a list of weird and wonderful conditions which will make you think 'Oh yeah, I remember, didn't George III have that'. Explore a bit – there are discussion groups, patient support groups, direct links to the world's major centres in whatever it is you're talking about.

There are also links to some of the alternative medicine gang, whose case, it has to be said, in some instances, can be quite persuasive.

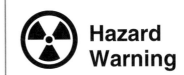

Hazard Warning

Pay attention now – you have to get the address right. No gaps, no full stop at the end and the _ sign is an underscore not a dash.

And did you have to punch in your General Medical Council registration number to get access to all this information? No. Anyone can do it. In fact, the government has laid out its stall quite clearly here in that everyone will have open access to the whole of the National Electronic Library of Health.

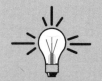

THINK BOX

Half of all patients are above average intelligence and 10% are brighter than doctors. Once folk who've got some of these conditions get wind of what's available on the Web, you can bet your bottom dollar that they will get to know these sites inside out. What is it going to do to the traditional way of doing business when the patient knows more about a condition than the doctor?

EXERCISE

 Take maple syrup urine disease as an example and pretend you don't know anything about it (probably not too difficult, if we're being honest). Now pretend you're a patient with access to the Web: http://www.msud-support.org/ (the – is a dash in this one, not an underscore), and work it out for yourself.

Will you get more information from your local GP/hospital or the Web?

Design an alternative care pathway for maple syrup urine disease.

What are the implications of this for revolution of the delivery of healthcare?

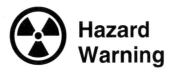 **Hazard Warning**

Viagra is wonderful stuff which will undoubtedly transform the lives of many couples whose relationships are marred by erectile dysfunction. But fast on the heels of its approval by the US Food and Drug Administration (FDA), a number of sites appeared on the Web selling 'sounds like' alternatives to trap the unwary. Names like 'Viagro' and 'Vaegra' that were not at all like the real thing. The Internet is notoriously difficult to regulate and many regard this as one of its main strengths – so in amongst the contributions of the 'Good' there are also certainly many contributions from the 'Bad' and the 'Ugly'.

Apart from the quality issue there is the question of information overload. There's so much stuff on the Web that you have to scroll through page after page of anecdote and trivia to get to the good bits.

There are a number of medical quality search filters that can help. They do all the hard work of establishing some measure of quality, surf the 'net for medical oriented sites, bless the good ones and filter out the rest. Two such sites are Omni (http://www.omni.ac.uk) and Health on the Net (http://www.hon.ch/).

EXERCISE

 OK, you've played with the Web and you have some idea of what it can do. Now put some thought into whether it's worth setting up your own website. Bear in mind that in the next few years, Web and TV technologies will merge so that most of the population will have direct and easy access to the Web through their TV. Also remember that you can easily provide links from your site to other sites that you think are reliable and may be useful to your team or patients.

- What are the pros and cons for you and your patients of having your own website?

- What information and links would you have?

- What about letting patients make their own booking via the Web?

EXERCISE

 Make your own website.

Here's a tip or two. Microsoft Word 97 let's you make a webpage and there is a neat little wizard to help you do it. If you want to go to the next step, try a piece of software called Web-Artist, by Sierra Home Software, available from http://www.sierrahome.co.uk It is not expensive and is the software Roy used to make his site – if he can do it anyone can.

If you are looking for a host for the site, go shopping in Tesco or Dixons and they will give you Internet connection software and space for your website, for free.

Remember, the most important thing about having a site is that people can find it. So, be sure to enter your site address on some of the big search engines, such as Yahoo and Loco. Go to their sites and there is a little button for you to click and get onto their directory.

Be sure to choose the right words for people to search under. Don't just put 'St Blogg's Hospital'. Put 'St Blogg's Hospital, telemedicine project, change management, information technology, bunions' or whatever the sector is that you have whizzed with your TMed project.

The hard work is not over when you've made the site – make sure you keep it updated. If having a good website sends the right message about your organisation, an out-of-date one has completely the opposite effect.

Finally, include your email address for feed back.

P.S. Look at Roy's site and you'll see you can buy his books from an online vendor, Barnes and Noble. He's not silly as B&N pay him 7% commission for having their ad on his site. Try http://www.free-services.com and see what you can find. Can you make your website an income generator?

Next funny phrase

VTC. Now this starts to get sexy. We've only been talking about ordinary phone lines so far and the anoraks start to take interest at this point. VTC stands for 'Video Teleconferencing'. This is where two people, miles apart, can look at a TV screen and see a fuzzy head and shoulders picture of each other – in real time. Wow!

Oh, so cruel and cynical! Well, the technology has improved quite a lot and the view is a bit clearer these days but still very variable. For all practical purposes you need to consider VTC at three levels.

The first level is for the cheapskates who don't want to shell out on any more kit or pay any more for their phone bill. There's something for them. They can buy software packages from the local computer shop for less than £50 that will allow them to VTC across a standard phone line with someone else at the other end with the same package. We're not going to tell you what to get because a new faster, better, cheaper one comes out every couple of weeks – so just ask the man in the shop.

 TECHIE STUFF

As you know, we've put this in a box because we don't want you to get too keen on the technical bits because your partner will leave home and your granny will buy you an anorak for your birthday. However, you do need to know just a little bit of techie stuff at this point.

Bandwidth is the size of your phone line, or rather it is a measure of how much information can be pushed down it in a second. The bigger the bandwidth, the greater the information flow and the better the picture. It is measured in KBps (kilobytes per second) – the more the merrier and the more it costs.

Standard phone lines are made of copper and are very slow. On a good day you can only get 33 KBps down one of these and hence the image is poor and movement appears jerky. Call charges though are at the standard rate.

It can actually be cheaper than a normal phone if you use the Internet. Some of the packages can be used across the 'net and so you can have a fuzzy VTC with friends in Australia, or anywhere else they may be, for the cost of a local call to your Internet service provider.

Far better to use level 2 – the Integrated Signal Digital Network (ISDN). You may have seen the adverts on the TV. ISDN 2 works at 128 KBps and so the picture is much better. But there is a catch, there always is – it costs more. Not too bad though.

It actually uses the same copper wire but the man from BT will come round and put a fancy box on the end of it which will allow much more information to be pushed down it. You'll also need another box called a TA (terminal adapter, should cost £200 but watch out for a BT charge of around £500) which decides whether an incoming call is a phone call or a VTC and flicks switches accordingly.

You can do a lot with ISDN 2 and consultations that do not need fine detail, such as psychiatry, can be done very nicely across it.

You can do a lot with ISDN 2 and consultations that do not need fine detail, such as psychiatry and general outpatients, can be done very nicely across it.

As well as getting the man from BT around, you will also need to get another box with a screen to actually do the VTC – you obviously can't do it down the phone. BT has just the thing and will sell you one for £5000 upwards.

Far cheaper though, is to buy a VTC board for your desktop computer (currently less than £1000) and pop it in. It is nothing like as difficult as the techies would have you believe. If you can read a set of simple instructions you can probably do it yourself, or if you can't you'll know a man who can. Some new PCs come ready equipped with a VTC board.

Call charges are twice the standard rate because you are running two lines. Incidentally, if you go down the desktop route you can also use the ISDN line for surfing the Web at the speed of light, as well as take phone calls and faxes at the same time. Saves space and is much more convenient to boot.

For the really discerning who want close to TV quality, ISDN 6 works at 384 KBps and is terrific. Of course, the call charges are three times those of ISDN 2 and six times a standard call – getting the hang of it? You may need ISDN 6 for such things as neurology clinics where you may need to see a fine tremor for instance.

Whatever you choose, make sure the technology matches your need.

 TIP

Getting the most from your bandwidth

With a little attention to detail you can get a much better quality image out of the available bandwidth. VTC does not work like the telly. When you watch Coronation Street in the evening after a hard day at the office what you actually see is hundreds of pictures being transmitted to the comfort of your front room every second. Lots of complete pictures.

For example, when Jack Duckworth is seen standing at the bar of the Rover's Return pulling a pint, he is moving but all the bottles on the shelves behind the bar are stationary. The TV picture treats Jack and the bottles exactly the same and *refreshes* the whole picture constantly.

VTC would treat Jack and the bottles differently. As the bottles are static that part of the picture will not be refreshed; Jack on the other hand is moving and the changes in his image are transmitted as they occur.

So if Jack were to keep his mouth closed and keep *still*, then no new information will be transmitted until he just can't contain himself any longer.

So the three VTC lessons from Jack Duckworth are:

1   A plain background uses up less bandwidth to transmit and saves capacity for the important part of the picture. Try to avoid a white background though – a pastel blue is better.

2 Keep motion down to a minimum. For example, advise participants not to wriggle about and wave their hands around – it is possible to talk without using your hands. The greater the motion, the greater the change and the greater the amount of information that has to be transmitted. As you get close to capacity, the picture will break up into little squares called pixels. If that happens then stop and let the picture catch up.

3 Where possible, use head and shoulders views. If you do this, it keeps the hands and feet and general fidgeting out of the picture and so out of the bandwidth equation.

Wondering what system to buy?

Broadly speaking, as we've already discussed, there are the bespoke systems on wheels (£5000 upwards) and the boards you fit into your computer (£1000 there or thereabouts). There are quite a few of each on the market and within each category they're all pretty much the same – price is often the key determinant. However, some systems allow for a small square in the top right-hand corner of the screen that displays the image you are transmitting. This is a helpful reminder that you are 'live', so don't pick your nose or do anything else disgusting.

 TIP

While we're at it here's another little tip to help you along. Think about where you sit relative to the camera. If you sit too close, the tendency will be for you to look at the other person on the screen which means that your VTC partner will have a nice view of the top of your head.

Sit far enough away from the screen to enable you to look at the camera and screen together. The little square in the corner will help.

Multi-point VTC

If you think that's sexy, it gets even better because with the right kit you can VTC with up to 32 sites simultaneously – if you want to do that sort of thing. It starts to get expensive but so does getting 32 people to travel around the country to meet up in the same room.

The system is called 'multi-point VTC' and requires a special bit of kit called a multi-point bridge that costs loadsamoney. So, it's time to start thinking carefully about costs *vs* benefits – you know, business stuff. It may be that the capability is very attractive to you but will you use it enough to justify buying the kit and appointing someone to actually do all the co-ordinating, the scheduling and all the rest of it? If so, go do it.

If the numbers don't add up, never fear – the man from BT may still be able to help. He will arrange a multi-point conference for you and your friends on one of their machines – at a cost of course. It works like a conference call using a telephone and they only bill you for the call charges and for the use of their bridge. You use your own VTC kit, you all dial in to a single number and BT provides the multi-point bridge, the co-ordinator and generally takes care of the rest.

Multi-use

You can always use VTC for more than one thing of course.

With sexy, expensive kit like this, it's important to make sure that you get the maximum benefit from it. That means thinking about using it for more than one job and regarding it as a two-way tool. You may even be able to rent it out to other groups and make a few bob on the side.

Mature systems in the United States have got this off to a fine art. VTC TMed systems used to deliver healthcare to remote communities have become community assets. They use the same system for tele-education, tele-legal and tele-anything else you can think of. Doctors and nurses get their continuing medical education down it – the possibilities are endless.

EXERCISE

 You're used to thinking outside the box now.

Try doing it with VTC. List instances where the cost of VTC TMed might be outweighed by the benefits for your organisation.

Assuming you had a VTC system in your organisation (with and without a multi-point capability), what other things could you use it for?

The X files

Telemedicine and X-rays combine in a brave new world and delight us all with a new word: teleradiology (sometimes called computerised radiology (CR) just to confuse the unwary). Never heard of either? Well, prepare for a shock. This is one segment of TMed that has already really gone somewhere. The gurus acknowledge that it's 'mainstreamed'. In plain English, caught on.

In practical terms it means that any radiologist or hospital considering buying a new X-ray machine will actively consider purchasing a digital, rather than the old style, wet film, system. Yes, even in the UK. A digital system allows for the more efficient storage and easy retrieval of X-rays and, more importantly, will allow the X-ray images to be batted around a hospital at the push of a button (and even seen in two places at the same time), or sent to GPs or sub-specialists over the Internet. Both these characteristics have huge implications.

Peace has broken out

At the heart of these radical changes to the wonderful and wacky world of the X-ray is the fact that, for once, rival manufacturers have decided to talk to each other – in the name of giving the customer something really useful. Instead of being at war with one another in the highly competitive world of medical-imaging, they sat down and talked to each other and to their customers. In fact, it was the Docs who drove it, under the auspices of the Radiological Society of North America (RSNA)

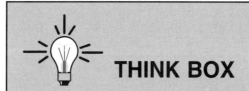

THINK BOX

Generally speaking, if you put three IT equipment manufacturers in the same room, you'll get five opinions and a fight.

The digital imaging people seem to have achieved a miracle – common standards!

In consequence, they arrived at something called 'common standards.' These standards are known by the acronym 'DICOM' meaning 'Digital Imaging and Communications in Medicine'.

'Never mind the tech-speak, what does it mean?' Well, since you ask. The result is that systems can talk to each other and pictures can be sent from one place to another without it becoming a major techno-drama.

An added bonus is that because the images are digital (that means that the gradations between black and white are turned into a mathematical formula and sent as a series of ones and zeros), they can be enlarged, manipulated and generally tweaked.

Most radiologists agree that digital X-rays now provide a better image than the old wet film system. Now there's a first! Professionals agreeing! Just joking.

PACS

As always, every silver lining has a large black cloud surrounding it. In this case it's PACS '**P**icture **ArC**hiving **S**ystem'. (If you are wondering, they had to put the C in so as to prevent confusion with hospital computer systems called 'Patient Administration Systems' (PAS).) Anyway, the only downside with PACS systems is that they are really, and we do mean really, expensive but they are the hub of the whole thing. The PACS is a huge data management system which does all the storage retrieval and transfer of images and although they are expensive, any Chief Executive or radiologist who has one would rather go and watch England play cricket than let you take it away. One day (in say five years), every hospital will have one.

Anyway, apart from better pictures there are also some less obvious benefits.

Conventional film is heavy and if you want to archive it, it needs to be kept in warm dry conditions. This means heavy-duty shelving, concrete floors, heating and ventilation systems. Digital images don't.

What folk often don't realise is that conventional X-rays can't be copied, at least not cheaply, meaning that an image can only be seen at one place at any one time and can't be seen at all if it's in the boot of the consultant's car.

It also means that if you stand a coffee cup on them you can easily damage them. And, as Roy will tell you following his recent 'incapacitation', X-rays can get 'lost'. In the US, a hospital passes its inspection if it can find 45%! – where do the rest of them go? Digital X-rays on the other hand, are 'virtual records'. The original is stored in a PACS, a computer's memory or on a disk. Therefore it is unlikely to be damaged and multiple copies can be syndicated for conference and second opinion purposes. They're hardly ever lost (and you can print out a hard copy too, if you really want).

Storage is even easier as the digital image can be compressed and millions of X-rays can be stored using relatively little computer memory and even less floor space.

Bad news for the shelf and concrete salesmen . . . sorry folks!

Here's a good question: ask radiologists how long it takes them to read routine chest X-rays. They will all probably tell you, with a certain amount of pride in their voices, 'about a minute or so'.

Oh, pride cometh before a fall!

Next question: 'Why then', you reply, 'does it take two days (if you work in a hospital, seven if you're a GP) to get the damn report back!' The answer is because it's all done by paper.

EXERCISE

Have you ever been into an A&E department in the middle of the night and had an X-ray taken of something that's worth your while turning up in the middle of the night for?

In every hospital in the land, even in the famous and the big, that X-ray will not be read by a grown up radiologist for 24 to 48 hours. With the best will in the world, the junior Docs who are tired and working their socks off in the middle of the night, might make a mistake. Some evidence seems to suggest they get it wrong in about 5% of cases. Is this good enough in these heady days of risk management and clinical governance? Can we do better? We sure could.

Using what you've just learnt about TRad, design a TRad network for A&E departments in the UK.

OK, not the UK. Start with your Region and work up! Think 'hub and spoke'.

Making a note of this

We accept that there will be the purists amongst you who will say this next bit has nothing to do with TMed – maybe you're right. But the next bit is featured in the NHS IT strategy and for that reason it is included. Also, if you think about it, it is at the heart of some of the major changes that TMed can deliver.

It's all about the 'Electronic Patient Record' (EPR).

 So, if you don't want to know anything about the EPR then flip over the pages and find a section that takes your fancy. We won't be offended.

Why include EPR in a book about TMed? The answer is, done well, the EPR will provide a pivot point for a lot more technologies to come together – and that includes mainstream TMed.

Given the welter of technology that surrounds the electronic recording of data and words (optical character recognition and the like) and the fact that other industries are making regular use of these technologies, why does the NHS make such heavy going of the EPR?

There are two main reasons.

Number one, the Docs don't like it. Why? Although they understand that patient records belong to the Secretary of State for Health and not them or the patient, they have still come to regard the records as 'their' records and a personal and private note of their observations.

Some so resent the fact that a patient record might be accessed by a third party that they resort to ridiculous white collar, guerrilla tactics such as poor handwriting and silly acronyms. Those days are disappearing. No longer will the A&E SHO be able to discharge a drunk in the middle of the night with a simple eight letters 'PAFO, TTFO' (P****ed And Fell Over, Told To **** Off).

Patients can now demand to read their records, and risk management issues will require a clear written note of what has occurred, been diagnosed and the proposed course of action as an essential part of a doctor's defence in a medical negligence claim. Many claims against the NHS are lost not because the staff did not do something, but because there was no record that they had done it.

Number two, the law. Just recently the rules surrounding the need to keep a written record have been addressed and brought into the information age. Previously it was a requirement (by statute) for a written record of all patient encounters to be kept, so that 'get up and go' doctors who wished to move to a digital or an electronic patient record, had to keep two sets of records (or else fall foul of the rules). A useless duplication of effort that was a disincentive to all but the real 'tele-electro-digital' pioneers.

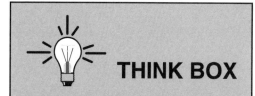

THINK BOX

The NHS paper on IT strategy recognises the need to move away from written records as soon as possible, and it is a stated aim to be wholly digital within seven years.

The NHS IT strategy recognises the need to move away from written records as soon as possible, and has the target of being wholly digital within seven years.

Number three, what goes in it? It is fair to say that the technology to do EPR is dead easy. Banks securely transfer records all the time and we don't bat an eyelid – and that's money! Far more important than people knowing about our piles. The real drawback is that the Royal Colleges can't decide what data should be included as part of the minimum data set, and also what shouldn't. It's not just our Docs – the ones on the other side of the pond are just as bad, except they are divided along State lines as well.

This is all part of the general smoke screen surrounding technology and it will prevail in the short term. But the stakes are too high for it to last much longer and the word from inside is that the EPR will be with us within two years.

But they'll never do it, it'll mean using keyboards and things

Yep – how to complete the record is the other big challenge.

Users of kit such as the Palm Pilot and the Psion 5 will tell you that handwriting recognition software is good but not fool proof. A record keeping system for something as sensitive as a patient record has to be really good. It is only very recently that technology has provided software that might meet the requirements of applications such as patient records. The latest is one called a

'Crosspad' that recognises the Doc's handwriting so that when he or she fills in the diagnosis box it is automatically ICD coded there and then, at the bedside. Wow! And for starters, Crosspad is already being integrated into the best A&E software packages. (For more see www.cross-pcg.com and www.hass.com.au)

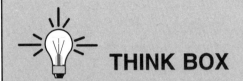

THINK BOX

Just think for a moment about the huge implications for managers, clinicians, public health Docs and the dinner lady, of knowing what is coming in through the front door of our hospitals   in real time! You never know, the system may even start to work.

What are the other options?

Next is inputting data through what the gurus call 'tick the box'. Here a labyrinthine critical path of questions is devised so that the Doc can tick the appropriate set of electronic boxes that reflect the patient's history, their condition, the diagnosis and suggested treatment and outcomes. This is complex, time consuming and seen as restrictive by some doctors. And, surprise, surprise, they don't all agree on what the questions should be and what the question pathway should look like.

Next? Well, 'touch screen' technology where a similar protocol-based critical path is presented to the doctor onscreen. The doctor makes the selection by touching the screen in the appropriate place. This is more user friendly but suffers from the same potential for complexity and restrictiveness.

What about voice recognition software?

It is getting really good now, to the extent that it has its own acronym – 'VR', not to be confused with 'virtual reality'. The only drawback is that it has to get used to the user's voice. The more you use it, the better it recognises how *you* speak and it becomes increasingly accurate. It learns how you speak and the words you use. The gurus call this intuitive software. There, you've got a new acronym and a new word to show off with in one paragraph!

The problem with this is that in hospitals, doctors come and go. Short of issuing them with a personal piece of kit and being able to do something about the inevitable background noise (a predictable part of life in a busy hospital), it is probably a non-starter for now.

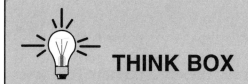

THINK BOX

In primary care and some quieter parts of a hospital, there is evidence that voice recognition systems will have a big part to play. We thought of writing this book using voice recognition software but the combination of a scouse and cockney accent, using the same PC, was all too much. However, we do have friends who use the system – John's mate, Eric, used VR to write his thesis on VR. They all say it is very good and he'll send you a voice written memo to prove it!

Currently, the answer to the data entry problem is 'horses for courses'. Radiologists in the peace and quiet of their reading room can use VR easily. Some are already doing it and have tailored their systems so that they just say 'normal chest X-ray' and the VR system automatically prints the Royal College of Radiologists' perfect description of a normal chest X-ray. VR is good for GPs too.

VR won't work for A&E though, at least not yet. Too noisy, too great a throughput of staff etc – so the top A&E systems currently use a combination of touch screen and Crosspad.

Shhh, don't tell anyone

Voice recognition kit is getting so good it will be included in the next release of Windows . . .

What else? At the moment there are no common standards for EPR, either for the records themselves or the methods of transmitting them. Where will the electronic health record reside? There are still a few questions to be answered and, we suspect, a few more to be thought of.

If you are really interested in EPR, try these websites:

http://www4.nas.edu/IOM/IOMHome.nsf/Pages/1997+reports

and

http://aspe.os.dhs.gov/adminsimp/pvcrec0.htm

They are US sites and are worth a visit but you know what websites are like. If by the time you get there they've changed or gone missing, don't blame us!

Let's look on the bright side

Let's vision what we could achieve if the NHS had EPR as standard.

Imagine a patient's complete record being available at all times. This would make registering with a doctor a lot easier and remove the need for the massive collection of filing cabinets cluttering up GPs' premises and hospital record departments – saving thousands of pounds on shelves and buildings.

It would mean no more risk of being run over by someone pushing a supermarket trolley full of patient records around the corridors of a hospital on the way to clinics and wards.

There would be nothing to lose or get pinched. A locum GP, visiting a sick patient in the dead of night, miles from anywhere could get instant access to the patient's history and record on his laptop, via the Internet. The obvious advantages are obvious. Obviously!

What about some of the less obvious ones? EPR could be a vehicle for 'store and forward' systems, avoiding the need to repeatedly write name and address details on in-house forms.

The printers will get very upset, but the NHS might save a few quid.

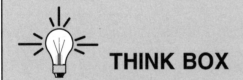 **THINK BOX**

Recently, Roy was in hospital for an operation on his leg. He had his name and details recorded eight times!

If patient records are digital and data based, they can be accessed in such a way as to give outcome measurements on adherence to clinical protocols and national treatment guidelines.

Common access to the same records means that there is less need to repeat tests and examinations, with the obvious attendant savings in costs and patient discomfort.

An EPR leads directly into electronic prescription writing. The obvious benefits here are the avoidance of prescribing contraindicated therapies and drugs, and the convenience of your medication being ready as you walk through the door of the chemists. Less obvious is the potential to help prevent fraud. Further down the list is the prospect of the prescription being generated electronically, sent to the pharma-warehouse from where it is despatched straight to the patient – Boots Direct. The high street pharmacy will have to stick to toiletries. (Have you noticed that pharmacists have recently been telling us how valuable they are as dispensers of good primary care advice – think they may be worried?)

EXERCISE

 Just be wild for a bit. Assume that all the privacy issues and security stuff has been sorted out, that the techies have got their act together and the country has, by and large, entered the 20th Century. What are the implications for the NHS of having a fully interfaced EPR? And remember that those who know about this stuff are confidently talking about it being a reality by 2001!

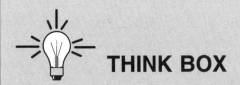

THINK BOX

You think we're joking about the Boots Direct quip don't you? Would we do a thing like that?

Check out www.planetRx.com It's an American Internet pharmacy. Honest. The concept is a bit Heath Robinson at the moment but it doesn't take too much imagination to work out what their R&D department is up to.

Here's how it works. You get your prescription from the doctor and send it to them in the post, or as a scanned image attached to an email message, or by fax. They then ring your Doc to make sure you're not cheating and then send your medication via Federal Express, next morning delivery and tracked by bar code all the way. The advantage for the patient, apart from them not having to go to the pharmacy? They guarantee they're 15% cheaper.

It's obviously not ideal for the acute stuff but what about all the asthmatics, hypertensives, diabetics etc who have to religiously troop up to their practice every month to pick up a repeat prescription, then march on down to the chemists, wait for an hour in a queue and buy half a dozen bottles of shampoo while they're waiting just to stave off the boredom.

Should the chemists be worried?

Here's what the pages look like – note the adverts for herbal medicines, big stuff in the US.

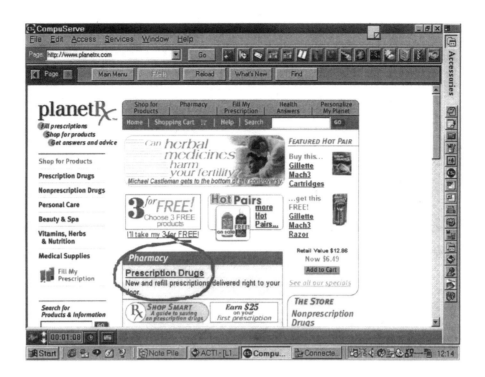

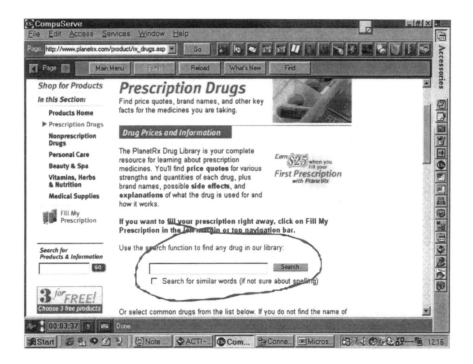

Section 5

So you want to do telemedicine?

Yes, yes, we know, you've had enough of the vision thing and the 'what not to do' thing, and all the rest. You just wanna get on with the job. It's worth reiterating as we start, that telemedicine technology is easy – developing a telemedicine service most certainly is not. And, as you will have gathered, introducing a telemedicine service is not just about rushing out and buying bits of nice new kit – although we do admit that that is the fun bit and that we like whizzy kit as much as everyone else!

We've said it before and we'll say it again. Complain we are hammering the nails in, out of sight, if you like but for the last time:

Telemedicine is a strategic decision.

It's not just about going out and buying a lot of neat kit.

And if you're really serious about getting it right, it is going to rule your life for some time to come.

It's always worth remembering the words of that great man of industry, Sir John Harvey Jones. He said:

'Planning is an unnatural process, it's far more fun just to do things and the really good thing about not planning is that failure comes as a complete surprise! . . . rather than being preceded by prolonged periods of worry and depression.'

So, having said all that, let's get down to it.

TMed *really* is all about planning and implementation, so here's what you do . . .

Twelve strategic steps for success

Check!

Step 1   Don't fix it if it ain't broke (*Work out exactly what you want to achieve*)

Step 2   Realise that technology will not be the whole solution – or possibly any of it (*Can you do what you want by just managing it better?*)

Step 3   Who's going to do all the work? (*Identify your Project Team*)

Step 4   Re-engineering 'outside the box' (*How will you do things differently?*)

Step 5   All aboard (*Engage all the stakeholders in the planning and implementation of the project*)

Step 6   Who wants what out of all this? (*Define the user requirement*)

Step 7   There's bound to be more than one way to do this (*Identify the technical options*)

Step 8   Nothing is going to stop you now. You wanna bet! (*Identify the barriers to implementation*)

Step 9   Define the clinical and business case (*For and against change*)

Step 10   Phased implementation (*Don't do it all at once*)

Step 11   Training, training, training (*That's training*)

Step 12   Ongoing evaluation and tweaking (*Is it right?*)

There you go. Dead easy. Rip this bit out too and put it next to the definition of telemedicine (*see* page xiii) on your notice board and we have the beginnings of a project.

It takes two to TMed, or is it tango?

It should be obvious but somehow we just forget.

Telemedicine has got at least two ends . . . obviously, right. So the great list of the 12 steps to the Telemedicine Hall of Fame just hit 24 because each one has to be done twice. And the answers to a lot of them are different for both so we can't even cheat and photocopy the implementation plan from end A, having added a liberal blob of Tippex and inserted end B.

It gets worse because end B is probably in a different organisation than end A and is almost certainly from a different 'level' in the NHS food chain, GP to local hospital for instance. Cultures will be different. The two ends are also separated by distance, which is sometimes huge. No point otherwise is there? Co-ordination, planning and meetings are going to be a bit of a challenge.

So before we start you need to put some thought into how you're going to manage this.

EXERCISE

Get together with the folk who you are planning to work with and work out how you are going to work together. Start by telling them to go out and buy a couple of copies of this book so you're all planning from the same toolkit (and no photo-copying it).

Both write down on this page what you have agreed to do

We won't bang on about this too much more, because it's really too obvious and we'll all get bored. But we may just remind you when it's important:

Remember it takes two to TMed.

OK, let's look at each of these 12 steps in more detail.

Step 1: Don't fix something that ain't broke

Define exactly what you want to achieve. What do you want to do and why do you want to do it? Before embarking on a TMed project it is important to define *exactly* what you want to achieve.

And, remember it is not a TMed project yet and may never be one.

There are two reasons for doing things differently, one is to fix something where the wheels have come off – big time – and the other is to improve a truly wonderful service. Let's be honest, it's usually the former but if you are looking to fix something that's broke you may as well go the whole hog and try and actually raise yourself above the hoi polloi.

Be a top dog and an example to us all.

So, what problem are you trying to solve or what element of your practice or service are you seeking to improve – and why?

Identify the factors you feel are important.

What are your core **vision**, **values** and **philosophy**?

EXERCISE

 Get the team together and work out exactly what you are supposed to be doing, what you're good at and where there is an opportunity to improve. While you're at it, work out what the constraints are in doing it right now.

Here are a few ideas to get you started – and remember no technology, at least not yet.

Factors	Importance out of 10	Constraint out of 10
Quality of care		
Quality of service		
Staffing issues		
Costs		
Over to you . . .		

Now go back and do it again, and be honest this time. What do you really want to do?

And if you think we're being pedantic, here's a story.

What did they really want to do?

A certain community trust offered an outreach, one stop breast cancer service in one of their community hospitals. The consultant surgeon visited weekly and read the mammograms and aspiration slides himself. He realised that although he was a pretty cool dude, he wasn't a radiologist or a pathologist and so he put the slides and films in the boot of his car and took them to be checked by the relevant specialist down at the big hospital.

So, why did the community trust want to get involved with TMed? They wanted to install a teleradiology and telepathology link – which didn't come cheap, and actually wasn't technically feasible at the time! Why? Good question. They said it was a clinical governance issue to ensure the quality of the diagnosis. However, research showed that the consultant was already right in 99% of cases and in the 1% of cases he wasn't right the patient was recalled within 24 hrs. So, quality wasn't really an issue.

What was the real reason? The truth is, they hadn't thought it through at all. And when they did think it through they realised what their real motive was. That was to support a vulnerable community hospital faced with closure.

So, let's ask the question again. Whadeiyeireallyreallywannado?

Another word or two about change?

Roy once met a NHS manager who complained that 'the goal posts were always being moved'. He reminded him that if things didn't change we could get by with a few administrators. Change needs managing which, as far as he could see, was the whole reason for this miserable being taking up space on the planet. He changed his mind about change. On the other hand, you sometimes come across managers who fancy they are good at change – they're a pest, too. If you've got someone who is good at change, get rid of them. Otherwise they'll always be changing things! Ooooh, such cynicism in one so young!

The NHS is always up to its neck in change! Buried in all the turmoil of change are some really good TMed projects. The trouble is, there is no mechanism to cascade what they do into the NHS. They are all a big secret.

Fear not. Hidden somewhere in the NHS is a secret and ugly band called the 'Telemedicine and Telecare Reference Group' facilitated by those wonderful people at the IHM. In a blinding flash of brilliance – for which steering groups in the NHS are not known – they decided on a revolutionary policy. A policy so unique it can hardly be written about.

They contacted a wide range of leading experts and asked their opinion. Fancy asking for advice! Well, they did it. They asked the top NHS gurus and their mates who knew anything about TMed what they thought were the top five things the NHS should be doing, using TMed techniques, by the year 2010.

Well, it turned out to be a waste of time. Everything the gurus suggested was already being done, somewhere. Just for the record, here are some of the things they came up with:

- Home monitoring of patients and self care
- A&E and community-based radiology with 'hot reading' of results
- Store and forward consultations
- Teleconsults and follow-up
- Emergency telemedicine
- Telepsychiatry.

No rocket science there. What do you think?

EXERCISE

Be a guru, or even better, get your team together and be gurus together. There is going to be a lot of teamwork in the pages ahead. Brainstorm and get everyone to list their top five things they think the NHS will be using TMed for by 2010 and send 'em all by email to John (navein@tatrc.org) for inclusion in the next edition.

By the way, 'brainstorming', what's that?

Brainstorming – here's how to do it properly

Brainstorming is the creative generation of ideas relating to a single topic. Such as, 'How could we use IT to speed up the arrival of lab results?'

The facilitator encourages every member of the group to come up with ideas that might solve the problem or address the issue. The deal is, all the ideas, however daft they may sound, no matter how irrelevant or silly they may seem, are written up on a flip chart, so that everyone can see them. No one comments on the ideas and nothing is rubbished or trashed.

Once all the ideas have been generated, contributors have the chance to elaborate on them and the group to evaluate their merit.

A lot of ideas will be crossed out but the betting is you'll be left with some interesting and innovative solutions – and faster results!

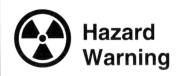

Hazard Warning

The facilitator has to make sure that ideas aren't trivialised or denounced.

If this happens members become reluctant to contribute, in case they are ridiculed or made to feel foolish. If that happens, good ideas may be lost!

 If that's tired your brain out – take a break.

Refreshed?

Now on to the last leg.

Planning for the way it's going to be

We have to be realistic here and accept that by the time we've got our act together; proposals have been around the houses; the Docs are happy; the IT folks will let you play; and you've scraped the funding together, we're not talking about TMed being open for business on Monday morning. Things will have changed and we suspect, changed big style. PCGs are now on the scene and some will become trusts fairly soon. Trusts and health authorities are merging and if all seems quiet on your patch now, it won't be long before some bright spark comes along and moves the goal posts. But we do need to plan and as far as possible, we need to plan for where the goal posts are going to be, rather than where they are now.

EXERCISE

Think about current trends in healthcare. The move to shorter bed stays and the shift towards primary care. And think about the trends that are operating on your patch. Where will your goal posts be in a couple of years' time?

Will these changes increase or decrease the need for a technological solution for your particular problem?

Don't forget it takes two to TMed. You need to do this with the team at the other end.

**Step 2: Be honest with yourself –
technology will not be the whole solution or possibly any of it**

Many of the things we think are wrong with the universe, world, continent, country, county, town, NHS, hospital or practice are often the result of poor process and management, not necessarily a lack of technology.

Even where technology is an important element of a solution it will only be a part of the whole. Changing ingrained old processes and persuading people to change to the new will be more of a challenge than introducing technology. Technology is easy but applied in the wrong situation it will make a bad situation worse.

EXERCISE

 Examine the problem you want to address. Consider whether it is a telemedicine issue or whether better processes are the answer.

Step 3: Who is going to do this fine work! Identify and resource the project team

Engineering TMed into your organisation is not a hobby. It is not a job to be done when the 'day job' is out of the way. The project team, if they are to succeed, must be small enough to be functional and have the sufficient time and resources to do the job properly.

The second thing is to persuade yourself that unless you wear your underpants over your trousers and can leap tall buildings in a single stride, this is a team thing. Quite apart from it being much more fun that way, it's also much more likely to succeed because the team feels that it is their baby too and they will keep you on the straight and narrow. Besides, a TMed project takes far too many separate skills and areas of expertise for any one individual to know it all. So get into hand holding, being nice to people, sharing and delegating. You'll be surprised. And don't just delegate the work, delegate the authority that goes with it and make sure success comes with a big pat on the back at the very least.

Who should be part of the team? All telemedicine projects need a clinical champion and a management champion working in partnership. The pair should drive the project with technical expertise in a supporting role only. Telemedicine projects should never be technically led. Don't forget a representative from the other end of the link.

 TIP

The clinical champion

Clinicians are very used to technology. Some parts of the NHS are a high-tech jungle. You can't move for bits of kit flashing and blinking and whizzing and things going beep.

But, and a very big **but**. TMed often involves a large slice of re-engineering what we do. Re-engineering is a nice euphemism. A nice euphemism for changing the way in which we do things – we've seen some examples already. Some Docs are not best known for welcoming change with open arms. So, a clinical champion – a Doc who is keen on what you want to achieve – is important. A clinical champion can often take other Docs with them and make implementation much easier. And they are very good at asking the 'pencil test quesiton'. What's the pencil test question? *See* page 10.

EXERCISE

 How would you identify a clinical champion? What would you need to do to get one on board?

Remember that the idea here is to use TMed as a tool to achieve or support the changes you want to make – your organisation should not be the tail wagging in response to the technology dog. But it's already becoming pretty clear that an average TMed project will mean change and a really good TMed project should mean lots of it if the technology is to achieve its potential.

So:

Is the 'boss' on board? Unless a move to a TMed-based service is supported, or even pushed from on high, it is likely to fail. Top level support is essential and as you are going to change the way things are being done, the boss has the need and the right to know. He or she will probably have a good few ideas of their own they're generally not as daft as they may sometimes seem.

There will be those who, for very good reasons of their own, may not be too enthused about what you are doing, particularly if it affects the way they work, or even their jobs. So you also need to make sure that if the 'neah sayers' try and use a back door approach, the boss doesn't trash the idea because he or she is not fully in the picture.

If you have a boss who is not exactly Einstein when it comes to technology, focus on the benefits to patients and the organisation to get them on board – keep off the whizzy bits, they aren't important and will only get him or her confused. And, in the NHS, where there is doubt nothing gets done.

EXERCISE

- Think about the clinical and managerial lead for your project. What qualities should they have in common?

- Think about the 'boss'. Describe how you would approach a 'boss' not known for their understanding of technology, and get them on board.

And don't forget the bit that everyone else always forgets at this stage – resources. Planning for telemedicine may be a part-time exercise in many projects but it is not spare time.

Resources mean time, kit, money, moral support, all those good things . . . And for each of them you should think of a number and double it. It always takes more time and effort than you think.

Dedicated project time is good. A fixed afternoon or couple of days where the whole team gets together to brainstorm (you know how to do that now), plan and set achievable targets.

TOP TIP

Email is a good way to bat ideas around. And don't spend days trying to get a document perfect yourself. It's much more efficient to do a good first draft, do a spell check and then pass it on to someone else with a fresh eye.

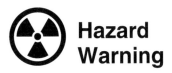

Hazard Warning

Spell check programs don't have idiot checks and if your spelling mistake actually makes another word, it won't show up – so don't rely on it. You won't find any in this book, and if you do it's all Roy's fault and he'll buy you a pint (if you can catch him!).

They'll never catch me John – here's one I spell checked earlier (RL):

I HAVE A SPELLING CHECKER
IT CAME WITH MY PC
IT CLEARLY MARKS FOR MY REVUE
MISTAKES I CANNOT SEA
I'VE RUN THIS POEM THREW IT
AND I'M SURE YOU'RE PLEASED TWO NO
IT'S LETTER PERFECT IN IT'S WEIGH
MY CHEQUER TOLLED ME SEW

EXERCISE

Work out the time, resources and timetable you will need to undertake the initial planning for this project.

Don't forget it takes two to TMed.

Stay in your lanes

We already know there are three parts to implementing a TMed scheme:

- the clinical bit
- the managerial bit
- the technical bit.

It is important that managers don't try and second guess the technicians; the technician doesn't try and do the manager's job and well, this is all a bit tricky.

Quite a lot of doctors fancy themselves as being a bit of a propeller head. They get bored being a Doc all day. You can understand it. For a Doc, the first time they diagnose measles they feel like Albert Schweitzer. After 3000 diagnoses, they must feel like a large gin!

Doctoring can be boring, dull and depressing, especially with all the paperwork and admin stuff they have to do. And these days people are even making them accountable! Whatever next! Not surprising they look around for something to apply their brainpower too. That's when they turn to management and become technicians. Dangerous!

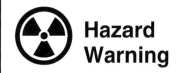 **Hazard Warning**

Doctoring can be boring, dull and depressing. That's why they look around for something to apply their brainpower to. That's when they turn to management and become technicians. Dangerous!

EXERCISE

 Consider your role as a project manager for an IT implementation. What management techniques would you use to make sure the players 'stayed in their lanes'?

Step 4: Re-engineering 'outside the box'

Pardon? Re-engineering 'outside the box' is guru speak for the old game we used to play as kids – 'consequences'. Here's an example: in the banking industry some benefits resulted from the introduction of hole-in-the-wall cash dispensers but far more came from the centralisation of services and the closure of small branches, so that now we have some banks with no branches at all and a 24-hour service. Smart, eh?

Telemedicine can be used to three different effects:

- It can be used to 'automate' what you are doing now – no points for this

- It can help you do what you are doing now differently – that's re-engineering and you get lots of points

- It can help you do something you can't do now, at all – lots of points for this too.

So how can we use TMed to change what we do?

 Make yourself a cuppa, put your feet up and consider these tales.

Pressing buttons as a lever for change?

Well, that's a nice mixed metaphor! This is really about using technology to bring about change and how, sometimes, technology solutions will bring about some unexpected changes and welcome windfall benefits.

A famous London teaching hospital had a problem. They were inundated with requests to investigate patients suffering with rectal bleeding. This requires a sigmoidoscope test but they had neither the medical manpower nor the real estate to take on any more. The answer was to establish a TMed link to enable a nurse to carry out sigmoidoscope investigations at a remote site. The images were sent live by VTC to the consultant in the main hospital – he 'oversaw' what she did and made the diagnosis. This obviously didn't save any medical time and in fact meant two people examined each case, whereas in the original model it was only the Doc.

One step backwards!

Over time the nurse became so proficient that the consultant started to fall asleep over the Times crossword! Now the consultant no longer looks over the nurse's shoulder – unless she isn't sure or there is a problem, and when that happens she takes a digital photo and sends it S&F. Marvellous.

Two steps forward

When the TMed link up was first designed it was an expedient way of getting more patients seen and solving a real estate and staffing problem. By the time the system matured it had resulted in a re-engineering of the service and introduced the concept of remote nurse-led sigmoidoscopy clinics.

You never know, they may even send the nurses round to GP surgeries next or even, dare we suggest, have nurse specialists working in the community as part of the PCG team. You never know, but it would certainly sort out the hospital waiting list problem.

EXERCISE

Yeah, we know you're having a break but if you can just juggle the coffee mug for a few moments and jot down the advantages of this re-engineered system for the patient (clue, there's lots) *vs* the old one (clue, not very many at all).

While you're at it, do the same exercise for the hospital, the PCG and London Transport.

Have a heart

How about this for a story? Did the consultant use TMed to bring about some sneaky change – he says he didn't, what do you think?

A major A&E department in the Midlands had a problem – don't they all! This problem was that all the patients with heart attacks were taken to A&E rather than to the coronary care unit which was located on another site. This was no good for patients as it incurred a delay in transferring them to what the gurus call 'definitive care'. It was also costly for the system as it invariably involved two ambulance trips.

So, our hero went to the cardiologists and said, 'Can we send all the patients direct to you?' 'No', they said, 'we've been doing it this way for years and there is no need to change'.

Undaunted, our hero then established a TMed link from the ambulance to his A&E department, so that the paramedics could transmit ECGs ahead for an opinion, prior to the arrival of the patient at the department. He then went back to the cardiologists and told them that he had a wonderful new TMed project and explained to them what it was.

'You can't do that', they said, 'You are just A&E weenies, what do you know about ECGs? You have to have the hospital end of the link in the coronary care unit!'

'Fine', said our hero, sensing he was on a winner – and so it was done.

What happened on the day of the race?

Well, the paramedics were called to scoop up a heart attack victim and radioed ahead to the coronary care unit sister and said, 'We have a male patient aged 55 who smokes 40 a day, has crushing central chest pain radiating and is sweating profusely. He looks really awful and we are just about to transmit the ECG'.

Sister said, 'Don't bother sending me the ECG, just send me the patient!'

The TMed link has never been used since! Our hero's plan was to change the process in the hospital – to send heart attack victims straight to the coronary care unit for the definitive care they needed, by-passing the risks and delays of going to A&E first. Sneaky, eh? There's more to this TMed lark than you think, isn't there?

EXERCISE

Consider some of the clinical practices where you work. Are they all ideal? Look again at your plan with a re-engineering hat on and think about how things can be done better. Now, what changes do you want to bring about that TMed can provide the lever for.

And,

What would be the jackpot bonus you could bring home if you did it?

 TIP

Is it going to work and do you really, really, really need a TMed solution? Talk it over with your team – enthusiasts and sceptics alike. What's the potential for a TMed-led solution? Yes, involve everyone including any leading members of the National Association of Technophobes and Sceptics who may live in the dark corners of your organisation. Winning them over may be crucial to success – so start early. On the other hand, they might be right and you need to know now!

You really, really do have to do this with your friends at the other end of the link – you can't re-engineer on your own, it's just no fun.

So, here we are at the end of Step 4. You know what needs to be fixed, you know what your constraints are and you have got the 'outside the box' thing down to a tee. All that remains is for you to convert that into exactly what you are going to do. This is what those fine chaps in the military call a 'Mission Statement'. And you're only allowed one mission – two means a split force and descent into certain failure.

Once you've done this bit, it is set in concrete. No veering off to one side or trying to fudge it if the going gets tough or something more fun comes up. Again, as the military would say, 'there's the target, give it lots of smoke and go for it straight up the middle'.

EXERCISE

☑ Write here what you want to achieve:

Our mission is to . . . .

. . . .

by doing . . . .

. . . . in order to

achieve . . . .

. . . .

. . . .

We are planning to use telemedicine because it will give us the following benefits . . . .

. . . .

. . . .

If you can't summarise the project in the above space, you need to do some more thinking about clear thinking.

Don't put this on the notice board. Get hold of one of the banner-making software programs and put it in letters two feet high across the top of the notice board and make everyone read it every morning.

Don't you just love planning? It gives you a warm fuzzy feeling that you might actually succeed.

> **Step 5: 'All aboard' – include all the stakeholders**

Technology frightens people. Yup, it really does. You've heard the toffs at dinner parties:

'Dahling', they cry, 'we've just bought a wonderful new video machine. Honestly, I don't understand a thing about it, we just have to leave it to the children to make it work.'

Don't you just want to reach for the butter knife and stab 'em . . .

And if you're so bold as to put technology and re-engineering together in the same sentence, wow!

So, you have to get them onside, or at least not offside.

If you plan to introduce a telemedicine service it is important to include all the stakeholders early. And, don't forget that that is likely to include patients or their representatives. Early involvement reduces fear and encourages owner-ship in the project.

Three important steps:

- Sell the vision thing
- Have the stakeholders help build the system
- Make sure they become the champions of the new processes.

 TOP TIP

Ensure that the enthusiasm of the entrepreneur is tempered with the practical considerations and natural scepticism of those who will use it.

EXERCISE

- Identify the stakeholders in your project and list them.

- Devise an approach that will ensure the early involvement of the stakeholders, so you can ensure that services and technology develop in parallel and are designed around their needs.

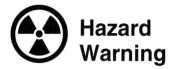

Hazard Warning

Believe it or not some people think that change in general, and TMed in particular, is a very bad idea indeed. What is really irritating is that they generally won't tell you that but will smile nicely and say what a good idea. Identify them early and smile back. Don't blame them, they can't help it and remember, they have mothers too.

Steering Committees

Steering Committees are a difficult call. If you play it right they can be a godsend, but get it wrong and oh boy . . .

TOP TIP FOR THE UNSCRUPULOUS

(Do not read this if you are the type who never parks on a yellow line.)

This is where your previously planned cups of coffee with the bosses start to pay off. Pop in to see the boss again and suggest that a committee would be a good idea – to ensure that everyone has input into the process and knows what is going on *blah di blah di blah* . . . and know that so and so (*your friend*) would be glad to chair it. Make sure that the forces of darkness are on the committee and have enough of a voice to be heard. Get the boss to endorse it and ensure that the real power rests with the Chair, who still remains, of course, your great friend.

TOP TIP

And raise the stakes. Get the idea in the local rag, hospital bulletin or even better, get the boss to bring his or her boss round to see what wonderful things you are doing and how important it is for the future. We're really bad at this sort of thing but it works wonders. Everyone wants to be associated with success and once they've nailed their colours to the mast they will make darn sure that it works.

Step 6: Who wants what out of all this? Define the user requirement

---

TMed is a tool, just like you need a shovel in the garden or a spokeshave in the workshop (*what's a spokeshave? Ed*). TMed can be seen as both a management tool and a clinical tool. So there must be three elements to this:

- What the clinical team wants

- What the manager wants

- What the technical support can deliver.

EXERCISE

Implementing TMed is a partnership. It is not technically led. Describe how you would develop partnership arrangements to ensure TMed delivers the expectations of all sides.

So you have your project team, you know what the project is aiming to achieve (mission statement – the thing in big letters above the notice board), you know what everyone wants and that the team is on board, and you've started to work on the problem of how to achieve it.

The next step is to define the user requirement.

What's that?

A user requirement is a statement of what the user wants the technology to do. It is *not* a technical specification. This is where the principle of clinical and management-led working with technical support comes to the fore.

Here's an example:

'We want a video teleconferencing capability which will link location X with locations Y and Z. We want all three to be on line at the same time and for the quality to be as good as a TV. We expect to use it for one hour a day and blah, blah, blah . . .'

Get the idea? Not a mention of a bit, byte, electron or even a plug. This is where the users tell the techie what they want.

EXERCISE

 Get the team together and brainstorm this through. *Exactly* what do you want the technology to do? It's a good idea to have the techie there too because he knows the options – but don't let him take the lead.

That's it then. On to Step 7.

> ### Step 7: What do we want to do here? Identify the technical options

This is all about supporting the user requirement with the right technical solution. Just to make life easy, there will often be several technical solutions. The team must consider the pros and cons for each. The gurus call it a 'benefits analysis'.

'Stay in your lane' is an important principle at this stage. It means stick to your role. Many TMed projects flounder because technical people try to second guess the needs of the clinicians or management or vice versa.

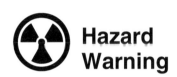

Hazard Warning

We've said it before and we'll say it again:

Stay in your lane!

The techies will be feeling a little unloved by now. The clinical folk, the managers and the team in general have had all the fun, and all the techie has been asked to do is to give a few ballparks. So let him have his day. Give him the results of your labours and let him get on with it. He is the expert now.

So, when you are driving a project, avoid a crash – stay in your lane!

Give your techie the time and resources to do a good job and be on hand to clarify any queries he may have. Agree a reasonable deadline by which they will come back to the team to tell them what the options are and the pros and cons of each.

TECHIE STUFF

Digital cameras

Digital cameras are pretty cool these days. You wouldn't want your wedding photos taken using one but they're fine for holiday snaps – and clinical photos. The surgical teams working in Kosovo used them all the time for their TMed link ups. And the cost is getting pretty reasonable too – you can even get one free if you buy the right computer.

Ah, we hear you say, for clinical photos it's obviously got to be the best. Wrong, a middle of the road one will do very nicely for what you need to do. As well as doing standard bumps, bruises and the occasional rash you can actually get a pretty good image of an X-ray on a light box or even a path' slide down a microscope, using a standard digital camera. Not the right solution if pathology or radiology is your day job but the military and Docs in Antarctica use it all the time.

The great beauty about digital cameras of course is that they produce a digital image rather than a film. No more trips to Boots in July to get last year's snaps developed before your August holiday this year. They are there instantly, and if they are not good enough you just delete them and take 'em again. And you can store them electronically, attach them to an email message (store and forward) and send them to whoever you like, in seconds.

Image quality

Instead of using films, digital cameras capture images on a charged couple device (or CCD – this is tech-speak. Don't ask us what they are but they seem to do the trick). These widgets convert the light into millions of tiny coloured squares called pixels – obviously, the more the merrier but anything over one million pixels will do. To give you an idea, a pretty good computer screen on high definition uses 800 000 pixels.

Range

The camera needs to be capable of long distance shots as well as close ups. Try a few close ups with the flash to make sure that the body of the camera doesn't cast a shadow over the subject.

Storage

Images are stored as files and compressed to save space. Many cameras have a number of built in compression options. Check in the manual to see whether the compression is loss-y or loss-less, i.e. do you lose image quality if you compress it? Try for yourself and see. We advise, however, that you stick to 'normal mode'.

Transferring data

Images are stored on cards of one sort or another. There are two types: Smartmedia (the smallest and lightest) and Compactflash (holds most images). Some cameras save onto a normal floppy disk or plug direct into your PC, which for your purposes is probably the most convenient. They're all pretty easy to use. You really do have to try to get a bad picture but if you do, you just delete it and do it again.

Back to work

Your techie, after a week or two (or a lot more if you're not careful) will get back to you with a range of options, the pros and cons and ballpark costs of each. This is broadbrush stuff. He'll probably try to blind you with science. He won't mean to but they do have a language all of their own and tend to treat you either like a complete barn pot or this year's Nobel prize winner in IT. In either case you're on the back foot. So . . .

EXERCISE

Go back and get your user requirement and list all the factors you defined down one side of a piece of paper, and make sure you include cost. In the next column put the range that is acceptable to you and get your techie friends to add their options along the top. This will form a grid called a matrix and once it's completed, all will become clear.

Having determined the major infrastructure pieces of the solution, it's time to get to the important bit. The bit you will actually use – what the gurus call the 'user interface'.

Define the user interface

It's got to be easy. Like the hole-in-the-wall cash machines, really easy.

 TOP TIP

However good your interface is, there should always be less of it.

We've already put some thought into user interfaces, touch screens, voice recognition software and all that sort of thing (*see* pages 50–1). Now you have the chance to come up with your wish list.

It is really important to get this right. If it's not user friendly they'll not use it, if it's too state of the art it may get too expensive, at least for this year. Here are some rules of thumb:

The two click principle: if it takes more than two clicks to do anything they won't use it. Anyway, getting processes down to two clicks for most things should be pretty easy for any software 'wirehead' worth his or her salt. *Make it a requirement.*

The seven Rs of making it *really* work:

1   Realistic – *this is the pencil test, again!*

2   Reliable – *needs to be reliable under the conditions it will be used*

3   Rewarding – *should make them want to use it*

4   Rugged – *make sure it will survive wherever it's going to be*

5   Really easy – *to use*

6   Reasonable cost – *for its functionality*

7   Routine – *must be used routinely; no point having a box which will only be used in an emergency because everyone will have forgotten what it's there for.*

Integrated into the work flow

It might appear obvious to you and us but how many places have you been to where there is a great big computer screen between you and the person who is looking after you? Doesn't happen with British Airways check in desks any more – their screens are built into the desk so there's nothing to block that 'have a nice day' feel.

Another example from the bad old days is the concept of telemedicine suites, where all the expensive kit was housed. It was always in some far-flung corner of the hospital because there was no way that telemedicine would ever be given any convenient location. Doctors had to walk miles to parts of the hospital they didn't even know existed – could you get them to use it? No chance.

Desk top, bed side, that's the answer. Make it easy. Make it bespoke. Make people want to use it!

Invisible

We're a long way from this yet but one day we'll get to the stage where you'll never again trip over a computer or a whole snake's nest of cables – because they won't be around. They'll be built into the fabric of the building or presented wirelessly, with only a screen to be seen. Telemedicine won't exist then either and they'll keep books like this in the archives of some dusty museum. Medicine will have absorbed it and the 'technology way' will just be 'the way it's done around here'. A long way off perhaps, but we might as well make a start.

 TOP TIP

Start thinking about security – that's the kit type not the data type. Most self-respecting thieves would not dream of nicking any computer currently being used by the NHS, but the sort of kit you are considering may well be very attractive indeed. So don't forget to include security specifications within your user requirement. Think about marking and 'lock down' systems and things like that.

EXERCISE

Decide what you want your user interface to look like. Pop down to Tesco, McDonalds or a modern bank and get some good ideas. Perhaps ask a patient or two. Now, design the user interface and divide it into 'must haves' and 'nice to haves'.

Ask your techie to cost them, just by way of a reality check.

Last but certainly not least

Define the service levels that suit you and that you can afford.

These are the standards you are going to lay down for your supplier. How often can it break down; how quickly will they fix it; will they do it on site or will it have to be sent it away? That sort of thing.

And realise that service levels can have a big impact on cost. How reliable does it really have to be? The techies, especially the commercial contractor types, can really do anything you want or at least will say that they can. If you want total reliability 100% of the time they'll give you reliability 100% of the time (well nearly) but they'll almost certainly put two complete sets of equipment in – twice the cost for a start and the whole thing will be more complex and therefore more likely to go down in the first place. Then they'll have a chap on call 24 hours a day to fix the one that's down – more cost.

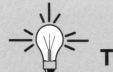 **THINK BOX**

Have you been down to Comet recently to buy a washing machine or fridge? They'll take good money off you and then ask you for more money to pay for a warranty so that they can come and fix it for you when it breaks down! Not much incentive there. A lot of suppliers make their money from service agreements and not from selling you the kit in the first place. The same goes for TMed suppliers. Try and come to an arrangement that puts the onus on the supplier to get it right. Consider a clause where you get a rebate if the system breaks but they get an extra x% if it beats all expectations. That should concentrate the mind.

 TOP TIP

Q   What's brown and looks good on a lawyer?
A   A rotweiller.

Nobody likes them but they do have their uses and can save a lot of heartache in the dark days to come. It's well worth running your service level agreements past your lawyers to make sure that the contractor cannot wriggle out when things go wrong. You can bet a big clock they'll have put it past their own lawyers to make sure that they can!

EXERCISE

Work out the service levels that are realistic for your purposes. Remember, if a system goes down before the team has got to the stage where it's indispensable, then they'll just go back to the old way and you'll have the devil's own job getting them back on board. On the other hand, get your techie to cost the various levels that will be available.

 Have a break!

Step 8: Nothin's gonna stop you now! You wanna bet!

Identify the barriers to implementation

Identify the barriers to implementation of the service. This sounds like it came straight out of the 'wet blanket department'. Well, it doesn't – it comes out of the reality drawer. The idea of identifying the barriers is to avoid driving into them.

Seriously though! No offence, but given the depth of tradition underpinning the NHS and a structure which has not, traditionally, been over keen to encourage co-operation, facilitate the shifting of workload or move resources, telemedicine is likely to come as a bit of a shock – because it does all of those things.

If TMed is such a good idea, why ain't we doin' it already?

Good question – let's look at some of the reasons, excuses, evasions, smoke screens, obfuscation and lies! In a world of innovation and change it is important to understand the forces of darkness – oh, scary stuff! Not everyone welcomes change and TMed is certainly about that. Resistance to change is natural, normal and understandable.

 Take a break. Here's a story that has nothing to do with TMed, but has a lot to do with institutional inertia and resistance to change.

What do you know about scurvy? Not a lot? Neither did the Royal Navy back in the old days. Next question: why do the Americans call anyone from the UK a 'limey'? The answers to both questions are interlinked.

Scurvy was a killer. In Vasco De Gama's voyage to the Cape of Good Hope in 1497 for instance, he lost 100 out of 160 of his crew to scurvy. Not such a good job being a sailor in those days, eh? By 1601 a chap called Captain Lancaster had worked out that the absence of fruit in the sailors' diet might have something to do with it. So, on one of his voyages he gave the crew of one of the ships citrus fruit, in the shape of limes, and gave the other ship none. The result was that on the control ship 110 out of 278 died from scurvy whilst the crew of the 'lime ship' remained healthy. Pretty good evidence-based medicine, eh?

However, the Navy was unmoved. Limes cost money! Not until 146 years later, in 1747, did James Lind revisit the scourge of scurvy. He sailed six ships around the world and gave the crews of each ship a different remedy – one of which was limes; molasses and rum being the two other contenders. Lind's method was to wait until the sailors got scurvy and only then did he give the crew of each ship one of the six remedies. Those who were only given limes to eat recovered in six days, the rest didn't until they were given them too. Game, set and match to the innovators, you might think.

Not so! It was nearly another 50 years before the Royal Navy adopted limes as a routine health supplement. The improvements in the health of Royal Navy crews are thought by some to be part of the reason why in 1805 we beat the French 20–0 at the Battle of Trafalgar.

And now you know why the Americans dubbed us limeys!

And while we're talking about the Yanks, they've had their moments too. This is a copy of a letter sent to President Andrew Jackson in 1829 by Governor Andrew Van Buren, no slouch himself and destined to become a later President. This was at a time when it was becoming obvious that new technology was winning out against the old canal system. It read:

'Mr President

The canal system of this country is being threatened by the spread of a new form of transportation called the railroad.

The Federal Government must preserve the canal system for the following reasons:

1 If canal boats are supplanted by the railroads, serious unemployment will result

2 Boat builders will suffer and towline, whip and harness makers will be made destitute

3 Canal boats are absolutely essential to the security of the United States.'

Read it again. All the old chestnuts are there. Have you met any destitute whip or harness makers recently?

Cheer up! Even some evidence-based innovation is difficult to implement. Back to work!

The feeling that TMed is not appropriate

Medicine is based on some fine traditions, one of the strongest being the doctor–patient relationship. The consultation is based around a face-to-face dialogue. A bit like the relationship we used to enjoy with a bank manager – remember them? Now we have cash machines and phone loans. Banking has moved on but, in many ways, medicine has not. Perhaps that's a good thing but customers have changed and become more demanding – and so will patients. We are right to be cautious and the intimacy of the consultation between the doctor and the anxious patient is something that needs careful consideration – but not all consultations are like that, are they?

Besides, TMed often gives the patient the opportunity to receive better and more timely care from an expert in another room, another town, another county, or even another country. Ask them which they'd prefer.

Clinical risks

If new ideas have risks, so do old ones – we just get used to them and work around them. People often question 'where is the evidence that TMed is any better than the traditional way?' Does it have to be any better? As long as it is no worse and brings with it the benefits of convenience and value for money, where's the problem? Well, there can be.

 Make another coffee whilst we tell you another story.

Some years ago, a psychiatrist who was very keen on TMed decided to manage his patients wholly by VTC. One of his patients was a female prisoner in a State Penitentiary, who was suffering from a psychological condition.

The Doc conducted a series of one hour-long consultations using real time video teleconferencing without ever meeting his patient in person once. Both he and the patient were very happy with how it all went.

All very well, you might say. The consultant's conclusion was that the patient's condition followed on from a period of abuse she had suffered as a child. She had 'lost' her childhood. His answer was for her to try and regain her childhood by reliving it through play and skipping in the exercise yard. The patient happily agreed with both the diagnosis and the treatment. However, on informing the prison nurse of his findings, she registered great surprise and said, 'Doctor, didn't you know your patient is paralysed from the waist down and lives in a wheelchair?' No skipping for her!

The problem was that the VTC screen only showed images of the patient and doctor sitting and from the waist up! The normal process that the doctor would have used was missing; he couldn't see the wheelchair and had no reason to doubt the patient's mobility. Whilst taking the patient's history, the issue never came to light. Had he met the patient face-to-face he would have seen for himself.

EXERCISE

What are the lessons to be learned from this anecdote? No prizes for saying TMed doesn't work! What are the elements that should be included in a televideoconferencing protocol to ensure the same sort of problem doesn't arise for you?

There are no technical standards

Yup, you're right. With the exception of the radiologists, who are way ahead of the game. Indeed, in the US they are using teleradiology to steal business from one hospital to another and from one State to another. The radiologists and the equipment manufacturers have forged an alliance, under the auspices of the Radiological Society of North America, called DICOM (*see* page 45). As a result, worldwide, all digital X-ray machines work to the same standards and have the same output. Any machine can work with any viewer.

At conferences, radiologists used to argue into the wee small hours about which was the superior image, traditional or digital? Now there is no doubt, digital is best

The same will happen for other specialties. Standards are not a mill-stone, they are a stepping stone. The early adopters of TMed will sort it out as they go.

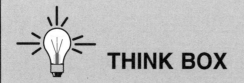

THINK BOX

Who should drive the standards process? The techies, the managers, the Royal Colleges? How would you evaluate standards and how will we know when we arrive at the best? Is the quest for technology likely to 'dumb down' standards or leverage them up? What do we use for benchmarks? Is the search for the best the enemy of the good?

TMed is too expensive

It used to be, but not so now! There was a time when manufacturers exploited NHS ignorance and were confused by NHS procurement dilemmas. The NHS's enthusiasm also added to the cost – an eager buyer often does not buy well.

The situation was exacerbated by the fact that there are three elements to the technical side of TMed:

• Hardware

• Software

• The communications link.

Each in itself involves a range of complex skills and each is a multi-billion pound industry. Each is also very clever – techies in each of the industries spotted an early opportunity in TMed and produced products that overlapped into each other's territory. More often than not, without asking the NHS what it really wanted. The consequence? A mess!

A one-size-fits-all approach emerged and little thought was given to what the real needs were. For example, did a system need a conventional keyboard? At the time most senior Docs were not really sure what a keyboard was. Today we all seem to be able to manage to get our cash out of a hole-in-the-wall bank. It's a computer called an ATM machine. It uses a keyboard. A keyboard designed to be intuitive, easy to use and do a specific job. You also get money at the end of it that may also help! With a TMed system you just get work.

Times have changed. A computer that once cost thousands now costs a few hundred pounds. Software that was once expensive is often free. Today everyone has a good idea of what the Internet is. And, most important, instead of the manufacturers of the three TMed components – hardware, software and communications – trying to infiltrate onto each other's turf, now they collaborate and ask the system users what they want it to do. They're no angels yet, but they're trying.

Products are emerging that are well designed, desktop based and inexpensive.

EXERCISE

List the attributes of a user friendly PC-based TMed system. How would you evaluate the needs of staff in deciding what the requirements are? What are the training implications?

Networking *vs* Competition

TMed is a powerful enabler of radical change. Sometimes that change means that not only will things be done differently, but it might mean they will not be done at all. At least not where they used to be done. That may have an impact on jobs, careers and empires. Since the reforms of the NHS in the early 90s, the NHS has become used to competing. The present reforms claim that competition destroys networking and the sharing of good practice. That may be true but hard evidence is hard to find. Nevertheless, what is certainly true is that change forces people to talk to each other. TMed has at least two ends and if you want to set up a TMed service you have to talk to the folk at the other end – not always easy. TMed is such a huge and powerful lever for change that it cannot be implemented without networking and managing change.

For some it will be a threat (or challenge), for others an opportunity.

EXERCISE

Imagine a locality with no district general hospital. Design a medical service from scratch. How many buildings would you need, how big would they be? Think about such concepts as GP specialists, nurse practitioners and the role of the pharmacist – plus, of course, the impact that TMed might have. Consider the impact on jobs and relationships with other professionals such as social services that better communication will bring.

If you haven't got a really interesting answer, you haven't been thinking.

Patient confidentiality is at risk

How secure is TMed and electronic patient data? A better question is, how secure is it now? A friend who is interested in TMed and electronic health issues and much sought after to give talks on the subject, tells of a neat trick. If he is asked to a hospital to give a talk, he always arrives early and makes a bee-line for the doctors' car park. Invariably he is able to write down the numbers of several cars that have patient notes or X-rays on the back seat. He says he never misses! This is the gold standard we are measuring TMed against. Ho, ho!

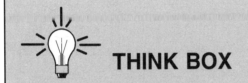 **THINK BOX**

Do you remember the time when a TV programme got hold of the medical records of the then head-lad of the BMA, Sir Sandy Macara? We bet you a pint they could still do it today. What could a determined journalist with a few quid to spend and a good private detective, get out of your place?

Modern technology is able to use all sorts of tricks and widgets to encrypt, anonymise and scramble data. The biggest danger is still the GP who leaves patient data displayed on an unattended computer screen. Or, worse still, gives their password to the receptionist! Perhaps even better is the GP who scribbles their password on a Post-It™ note, and then sticks it to the inside of their desk drawer.

Even simple encryption of a set of medical records would take a computer the size of Moscow a week to unscramble – and who is going to bother? If we all do the simple things, patients are better protected with modern technology than they are with paper. It's the process that matters. Keep it simple and keep it consistent.

Do patients care? Seemingly not. Although there is the story of a gentleman who spent half an hour in a minor injuries unit. Whilst waiting to see the nurse he was watching the TV in the waiting room. By coincidence, a medical programme was being broadcast. When he was called in for his examination the nurse asked him to remove his trousers so that she could carry out a VTC consultation, regarding his sore buttocks, with the consultant in the district hospital far away. The patient refused.

'Why?' asked the nurse. The patient replied, 'I'm not having my backside shown on the telly in the waiting room!' Moral of the story – explain to patients what you are going to do and they will usually go along with you!

EXERCISE

 Is special consent required from a patient about to undergo a teleconsultation?

What protocols would you establish for your own particular unit?

Does anyone have to bless it?

This is not as easy as it seems and it all starts to get a bit complicated – look over the page for a hint.

In general if a teleconsult is part of an
established telemedicine service, specific
written consent is not required.
However, if the consultation
is part of a trial then it is
wiser to obtain consent
from the patient first.

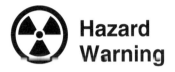 **Hazard
Warning**

When is a record not a record? Does a recording of a video tele-consultation constitute part of the patient record? Why tape it in the first place? We don't tape conventional consultations, so why tape videoconsultations? **So, don't do it**.

However, for training or audit purposes, it is allowed. But you do need to obtain specific consent from the patient.

Store and forward consultations, such as digital pictures sent to dermatologists, probably do form part of the patient record and should either be printed out and included within the paper record, or archived electronically.

EXERCISE

Here's a problem: if you are looking to record a tape for training and education purposes, how do you know you've got a consultation worth keeping until you've done it? You may have material that turns out to be of no value. In which case, can you destroy it? The answer is 'yes', but then the lawyers might well say, 'Ah doctor, why did you destroy this particular tape?' You know what they're like. *So there must be a tight set of protocols that deal with the issue specifically and form part of the operational procedures of the organisation in which you work.*

Devise a protocol under which teleconsults can be used in training videos, but can also be destroyed if they prove to be of no educational value. Consider issues of patient consent and awareness, the method of destruction and patient confidentiality. Who would need to approve the protocols and how would they be included in your operational procedures?

EXERCISE

Devise a set of protocols for store and forward systems that deal with the management and protection of the material. Who needs to approve the protocols?

EXERCISE

 Consider the barriers to implementation of your project. Take into account such factors as:

- The impact of the need for close co-operation
- Changes in the workload pattern
- Shifting resources
- Medico-legal, privacy and ethical concerns
- People factors
- Is this one change too many?
- The medical Mafia.

Give them a score from one to ten where ten is really hard but doable. Accept that there may be an eleven.

A word about matters medico-legal

Clinicians opposed to TMed will try and stop the show with a medico-legal argument. They will say, 'This telemedicine stuff is all very well, but who is responsible if anything goes wrong? Whose liability is it if the consultation misses something or reaches the wrong conclusion?'

They are likely to site an example of a GP referring a picture of a patient's rash to a dermatologist. Let's say the dermatologist gets the answer wrong, prescribes the wrong treatment and makes the condition worse. The unspoken questions are: because the dermatologist did not shake the hand of the patient, was it a proper consultation; was responsibility formally handed over to the consultant as in a traditional referral; and who is responsible for the patient's predicament, the GP or the consultant?

They're right of course, it does need thinking about. But medico-legal issues fit very firmly into the 'hurdle to be jumped over' category, they are *not* show stoppers.

The law is there to provide a framework for sorting things out when they go wrong and provide compensation or punishment where it is due. It doesn't matter whether they go wrong 'virtually' or for real.

It's a good time to remember that TMed has been practised for a long time and that there's nothing new about all this. GPs do a fair proportion of their work on the phone and they follow two Golden Rules:

- A teleconsult is not the same as a face-to-face consult

- If in doubt, *see the patient*.

TMed is not really around to improve quality of care, it's all about quality of service. It is a level of service above (sometimes way above) what is otherwise available but as soon as quality of care is compromised, then we must revert to Plan A: the gold standard, *see the patient*.

Different information flows during a teleconsult (*see* story on page 92) – different in both quality and quantity. All healthcare providers ask themselves each time they see a patient, even if sub-consciously, 'Can I safely manage this case, given the information and skills I have, or do I need to refer it on?'

Exactly the same goes for a teleconsult. If the clinician feels he/she doesn't have enough information or is unsure about the quality of the information on the screen, revert to Plan A: *see the patient*.

When in doubt, revert to Plan A: *see the patient.*

This principle also covers the other aspect of the same smoke screen, *who is responsible*? If the specialist answering a teleconsult is happy to make a recommendation given the information available, then he/she takes responsibility for that recommendation. If he/she is not, revert to Plan A: *see the patient.*

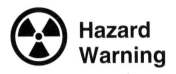 **Hazard Warning**

Having said all that, accept that this stuff is all pretty new and deserves additional attention to detail.

EXERCISE

Get together with your friends at the other end of the link and work out what the potential problems may be in doing business by TMed. Work out a set of protocols to protect them against litigation. Play Devil's advocate and try some 'what if' scenarios to make sure they work and, if you get as far as Step 10, take them out of the drawer and run them past the lawyers.

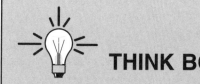

THINK BOX

At this stage although the barriers can largely be resolved as 'problems', think about how to do it and *if you want to do it*. Barriers can either be moved or overcome but don't be blinded by enthusiasm or macho-management. Do the barriers become 'show stoppers'? Even in the face of a strong clinical and business case, are there some barriers that should not be lifted? At least not yet.

EXERCISE

Define the difference between a barrier that must be jumped over, one that can be moved and a barrier that is best left alone. Consider circumstances where it would be unwise to proceed, even if you were able to demonstrate that the barrier could be overcome.

Are there any 'show stoppers' in your project?

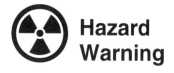 **Hazard Warning**

This is the first 'go/no go' decision point.

> ### Step 9: Grungy stuff – define the clinical and business case for and against change

Oh, sounds tricky and businessy and ugh . . .

Well it is – but it's got to be done, so let's get on with it.

First things first, it isn't rocket science – it can't be because we can do it! Let's start with the basics.

What is a TMed clinical and business case? The first thing to notice is that it's not just a business case. In our business there's more to life than just money, although it is important we grant you. So a simple definition might be: the clinical, managerial and financial justification for change using a TMed enabled service. That's the second thing: it's not just about measuring the cost benefit of TMed because that's not what we're doing. It's about assessing the impact of the whole change thing that TMed enables.

It measures what we are doing now, against what we want to do in the future and compares the two. The aim is to provide the justification for change *or staying the same*. The justification is based on the interplay between, and the relative importance of, the clinical, managerial and financial considerations. Again, it does not mean 'in purely financial terms'. That's why it's a clinical and business case, not just a business one – and clinical comes first.

Move a little closer to the page and make sure no one is looking over your shoulder. Here's a secret:

The insertion of technology into a system rarely saves money, at least not initially . . .

Now we've got that off our collective chests, here is the second part of the sentence:

. . . but TMed should *always* provide far better value for money, provide a better service for the patients and be more rewarding for the providers. They will all wake up on a Monday morning saying, 'Oh great it's Monday morning, off to work'.

Value and cost are not the same thing

Think of it in terms of the family car. Twenty years ago the average British Leyland (may they rest in peace) car was a tin box on wheels which took 17 people to make – and the radio was an optional extra.

Today a Nissan takes five people to make, it is packed with safety features, ABS brakes, airbags and the like, CD players come as standard, as increasingly does air conditioning – and, in real terms, it all costs the same.

Value may mean paying more in the short term in order to gain value in the longer term.

Even the government has cottoned on to this as a good idea through what it calls its 'spend to save' programme. Worth a visit to their website to find out how Whitehall's thinking is changing.

The other nicety in the title is the 'for and against' bit. We've got to be honest at this stage, it might just not be worth the effort – very unlikely but possible, so no cheating.

Who is the clinical and business case for?

The plan might be for a variety of interested parties. Just as books, magazines and newspapers take into account their targeted readership, so must the planner. Who reads the plan means adjusting how you write the plan.

 TIP

When you produce the plan put yourself in the shoes of the person who will read it and make the decisions to enable it to happen. Be honest with yourself. Does it make sense and can you deliver?

Is the plan for:

- people in your department, to give them a sense of direction and clarity

- your boss or a group of people who have the power to say 'yes' or 'no'

- people who will 'invest' or fund the project or service

- people who will use the service

- people who will work in the service and run it

- people who will give permission for the project to get underway

- . . . perhaps it will be a combination of all of them.

 TOP TIP

What will they need to get out of the plan to help them make a decision? Write your plan through the readers' eyes.

So, it's pretty obvious that what you are going to do has to be worthwhile or else there's no point doing it. Right? Now you have to prove it. No problem, you've done a lot of the work already.

Look at what you're doing now and cost it based on the factors that you identified as being important to you all the way back at Step 1 (*see* page 60). You even developed ways of measuring them too.

Now look into the future and work out what these costs are going to be once the system is in place. Don't forget that we are not just talking about dosh here. It's what really matters to you, your team and especially the patients.

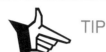 TIP

Don't overestimate demand or use of the service you are planning, and don't underestimate how hard it is to get a new idea off the ground.

Remember the 'S' in NHS and what it stands for.

Who is going to use this wonderful new service?

You may be surprised to learn that the concept of business planning and making the business case is relatively new, even to industry. It is a technique that is less than 50 years old. Only in recent years has it been adopted by the public sector – and in the NHS it has only been a regular management tool since the Thatcher reforms in 1990.

Words such as 'demand' never sat easily in the NHS dictionary. It is a word that is too close to the business community to be readily adopted by the NHS. Nevertheless, 'demand' or other words and phrases that indicate the extent to which services will be used, are a vital part of planning. Your plan is likely to underpin the development of a new service, so establishing demand is fundamental. If the plan is in the context of a start-up organisation getting some clarity about what it is offering and how it is to do it, then 'demand' as part of the planning formulae is indispensable.

EXERCISE

Identify who is going to use the service and what evidence you have that the service will be used. Define precisely the services to be offered and show how you will let people know you are offering the service. Is demand for the service seasonal, cyclical or constant? Finally, health is a high-tech business and today's good idea can easily be overtaken – demonstrate how you will keep ahead of the game.

EXERCISE

Take the matrix that you developed in Step 1 to measure your current costs of doing business, and repeat the exercise for when your TMed enabled service is up and running.

The difference between the two is the case *for* change. And don't be surprised if the difference is absolutely huge because it should be, especially if you have done the re-engineering thing properly.

Next add up the costs (initial and ongoing) associated with your preferred technical solution (you did that in Step 7), together with the costs of the change itself. Include such items as:

- management time

- training time

- the costs of the evaluation process

- capital depreciation of equipment

- ongoing maintenance contracts.

(Given the levels of savings that you have identified above, you may feel able to add in some of the 'nice to haves' as well as the 'must haves'.)

This gives what the gurus call 'the cost against change'. A comparison between the two constitutes a simple clinical and business case.

There, that was easy wasn't it!

Just one more thing! Having got the clinical and business case out of the way, you will also need to factor in both the 'pain factor', which is significant in any major change process, and the 'feel good factor', which will result following a successful implementation of a good project.

Have a break and once the caffeine starts coursing through the veins and you are thoroughly refreshed, start thinking about what you can do with the clinical and business case now that you've got it.

EXERCISE

 You've done the business case, so what?

Let's hope that the case you've come up with is nicely on the positive side (we always knew it would be). What are the implications?

List five 'so whats'.

We'll give you the first one because it's just too easy:

1   This is our justification for funding

2

3

4

5

Writing it up

We've already emphasised the importance of writing the plan through your readers' eyes. The boss and the bean counters will obviously be key players in this and it might be worth popping along to see them before you put pen to paper, finger to keyboard or even voice to VR microphone. Give them the gist of what you've found and get their feel for what buttons should be pressed hardest.

It maybe that the nice man (or woman) at the ministry has just announced a new initiative with funds attached that would fit the bill, or something is happening at Region that hasn't filtered down to the coal face. In the current climate, clinical governance, appropriate technology to modernise services and risk management are all flavours of the month, so if you can emphasise all of these and show that there will be a return on investment as well, then you should be on.

If you can hit all those buttons then chief execs will find it very difficult to turn you down and, if they've been on board from the start, they'll be knocking on your door saying why isn't it up and running.

A fully worked up clinical and business case, well presented, is such a rarity that they'll probably fall off their chairs. Be careful though, the only reward for good work is more work!

 TIP

Don't get beaten for the want of a bit of bulls**t. Presentation matters. People will always tend to judge the quality of the content on the quality of the presentation. May not be fair, may be daft, but there's no getting away from it. So add a logo or two, work on the layout, check the spelling (*see* Hazard Warning on page 70), consider a Powerpoint type of format rather than page after page of prose, and put it in a nice folder.

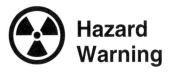 **Hazard Warning**

This is the second 'go/no go' decision point.

If the clinical and business case is not way over to the right, take up golf.

By now you'll be getting to grips with TMed and be familiar with guru speak such as 're-engineering'. But what do you know about management?

Before we get on to the implementation phase and the remaining three steps, there are a few things you may want to know.

If you do, read on. If not, skip on to the next bit.

Management for the aspiring telemedic

Who says management is difficult?

Management, like most things, isn't too difficult if you put your mind to it, but it does take a good dose of common sense, people skills and attention to detail.

You'll be well up to MBA standard if you've got this far but it's still worth just focusing on a few key areas before we face Steps 10–12. They are:

• Project management

• The management of change and

• Risk management.

Assembling a project plan flow chart

What's project management? If you can plan a holiday and make a shopping list, you can do project management. Think about where you are, where you want to get to and the steps along the way – that's called a project plan.

Topic	Action	Done, by when, by whom?
• Situation analysis • New information • National requirements etc	• Where are you now? • What are the issues? • Are there any national or other requirements you must take into account?	
• Key findings • Observations from the environment and trends	• What are the external factors likely to influence your success?	
• Opportunities and threats • The effect of the 'environment' • Relative importance	• Make an analysis of the factors and list them as threats or opportunities	
• Use opportunities and threats analysis to stimulate thinking about what is required	• Check capabilities – can you do it with the skills available?	
• Downside analysis • Anticipate problems and weaknesses	• Identifying the success factors • Are there any show stoppers?	
• Key issues • Opportunities and threats that are realistic and based on your strengths and weaknesses	• Situation analysis – what can realistically be managed?	
• Critical success factors	• What you need to do to achieve • Double check that forecasts are not over ambitious • What are your performance expectations?	
• Resource allocation • Expenditure • Staff • Logistics	• What do you need to do? • What do we have to put in? • What can we expect to get out?	
• Who to see to get support • Specific actions • By when? • By whom? • Review, check and monitor milestones	• Allocation of roles • Specific actions	

EXERCISE

 Guess what it is! Write a project plan.

Here's a reality check:

1 Starting a new project is never easy. Is it a real team effort or is it in the hands of the odd enthusiast? Is the project sound enough to outlast the people who start it up?

2 Do you really have the technical skills to make this work?

3 Is training required – have you allowed time for training and for the cost of training?

4 Do you have the skills to administrate the project? How can you be sure the enthusiast won't run away with the idea? Someone has to keep their feet on the ground and do the adding up!

5 Is the plan flexible enough to accommodate likely changes on the way?

6 Have you got the time to take another project on?

7 If you need to recruit, have you left time to get the staff?

8 Can you be sure the staff are available? Is there any kind of recruitment crisis in the professional sectors you will be relying on?

9 Is there wage inflation in the sector?

10 Are there any transport requirements for staff?

11 What's so special about this project?

12 Is there really a demand or is it just an expression of professional ego, or 'me-too-ism'?

13 Are you sure that the service you are offering is supported by potential users?

14 Will you be prepared to modify what you are offering in the light of patient experience or demand?

15 Is this the right time to introduce this service?

16 Are developments in technology likely to overtake you?

17 Have you spoken with potential users of the services? What is their impression of what you want to do?

18 How will you keep up to date with developments and demand?

19 Can you rely on the suppliers of your kit or consumables?

20 Are you starting with pump-priming money? How can you be sure you will be able to fund the service in the medium/long term?

21 Have you got adequate management information systems in place to keep abreast of what is going on?

22 Is the project sufficiently managed by a professional who is not emotionally attached to the project?

23 Is there full commitment for the project from others, such as peers, Board members, other service providers?

24 Are any special permissions, licences or consents required? Can you get them in time?

How many ticks have you got? If there are any 'crosses' think carefully before getting underway. Sort the problems out now, before you start.

Change, change, change – we've got more change than a bus conductor!

If you haven't yet cottoned on to the fact that TMed is about change, real, radical change – then you've either skipped a lot of pages (that's OK) or you should take this book back to where ever you bought it from and swap it for something more useful, like a book on Mongolian art.

Here are some thoughts on managing change.

When things change, staff become unsettled, they leave, their motivation drops and the performance of the whole organisation can go down the pan.

When that happens all kinds of other risks creep in. The team take their eye off the ball.

 Make a coffee and read through these pages. All the changes that TMed could bring about mean huge challenges and great opportunities – but a whole lotta risk.

This section is full of ideas and exercises to help you implement TMed changes where you work, without making it hard work.

They are all aimed at building a team that can face the challenge of change together and with the minimum of risk.

 TOP TIP

If you want to know more about team building in primary care, try *The PCG Team Builder*, also published by Radcliffe Medical Press, written by Gareth Davis, Bill Cain and, well, Roy is too modest to say!

A few words of wisdom to get you thinking before we start

We said at the beginning that you can flick around this book, take the bits that you want and generally cherry pick.

That's fine but it also gives us an excuse to say it again:

- Telemedicine is about enabling change, not just about buying widgets.

- Telemedicine is easy, developing a telemedicine service is not.

So, before we get on to the last steps to telemedicine heaven a few words about change management.

It's all change

Some TMed projects bring about change to the point where it might be better defined as upheaval! It could have an impact in every part of the organisation, on individuals, practices and for the professionals you work with. If you are responsible for a TMed initiative you are responsible for managing a change initiative – whether you think you are or not!

The risks in not managing the change element of a TMed project successfully are in the loss of motivation of staff, chaotic administration and the likelihood of errors occurring in the work of otherwise wonderful staff who are preoccupied with thoughts about their jobs, their future, even their whole lives – and you don't realise it!

Let's look at how TMed could affect the future delivery of services and take an easy example to see what the knock on effect of a seemingly simple idea can be.

Gimme some skin – dermatology

Let's get under the skin of the stories about dermatology. After all, we all know that dermatology is money for old rope and that dermatologists don't really want to see patients, they just want to see rashes – right? Say telemedicine and everyone's mind always goes straight to dermatology, coz it's dead easy, innit?

Or is it? There's a lot of truth spoken about it and a lot of nonsense too, so let's try and sort the dermis from the epidermis.

Dermatology is one of the areas of medicine where telemedicine can make an immediate and valuable impact. Do you know how long it takes, on average, to see a dermatologist in the UK? There are roughly 250 000 people waiting at any one time, with an average waiting time of around four months. And in Manchester the waiting time is over a year. Not exactly Kwik Fit eh?: 'We can do your big end on Monday Sir, but that nasty rash you've got, well that will have to wait until next May.'

Mr Milburn will not be pleased, and nor are the patients.

So, what can telemedicine do?

Let's look at what a traditional dermatology consultation actually entails. Faced with a four month waiting list, a GP will try and do it himself. Every GP knows that dermatology consists of two sorts of rashes – wet rashes and dry rashes – and that the treatment for wet rashes is to dry them and for dry rashes to put steroids on them. So that is, by and large, what they do.

Several months later, and after several increasingly fraught return visits to the GP, the GP admits failure and the patient finally gets referred to the big hospital. That process in itself is a bit of a song and dance when you think about it, with typists, secretaries, postmen and all the rest of the palaver of a paper-based system. Four months after that (if you don't come from Manchester), the patient gets to see the main man.

The patient will take a half day off work for the initial appointment and for a couple of follow-up appointments after that (it takes around 26 minutes of consultant time for each new patient). By the time the GP gets the letter back (again typists, postmen *et al.*), he's forgotten what the problem was in the first place.

We admit that we can be rather prone to exaggeration in making a point, but we're probably being kind with this one.

That's the way it is today, hardly what you'd call 'Health' and certainly not 'Service'.

Now let's look at it the new way

The patient goes to the GP with a rash. The GP knows that he has a responsive, reliable and timely referral service behind him, and so has no qualms at all about immediately referring a patient about whom he's unsure – that sounds like good clinical governance, doesn't it? He asks the patient the five GP dermatology questions, which we all know are:

- How long have you had it?

- Is it getting bigger?

- Does it bleed?

- Does it itch?

- What have you put on it so far?

The GP then sends the patient through to the practice nurse, as they would with many other conditions. They put the answers to the five questions on to an email message and takes three digital photographs: one close up, one far away and one oblique, and attaches them to the message. One click on the send button and it has gone and the GP didn't even have to touch a keyboard or a nasty rash.

The email message, instead of necessarily going to the nearest dermatologist, goes to the next available dermatologist. In fact, did you know that if you call the Freephone number for Swissair from anywhere in the world, your call will be answered in Calcutta? But we digress.

The teledermatologists reckon that they can deal with 85% of business this way and, of course, they don't have to be in a hospital. Why not work from home? Good concept. This is perhaps a good way to mobilise huge resources, medical professionals at home looking after young families. It's called the new NHS 'family friendly' policy. Could catch on for radiology and other specialties as well. No desks, no office, no secretarial support – all gone.

And an S&F consult only takes the dermatologist five minutes to reply because he/she doesn't have to be nice to the patient. It doesn't take the brains of an archbishop to work out that if it only takes five minutes of consultant time as opposed to 26 minutes, then the waiting list will disappear (along with the need for private practice – Oh, who said that?). And at the end of it you'll only need one-fifth of the number of dermatologists!

But there's more!

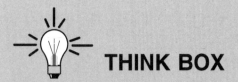

THINK BOX

By the way, any dermatologists reading this who think we've only scratched the surface of the problem, you're probably right. So please don't write to us saying we're picking on you because we are, and we are because it's too easy. But don't worry, you're not alone. The same principles apply to lots of other specialties too.

If this all sounds too easy – it is. But some dermatologists will say that they can't make a diagnosis without touching a rash and seeing a patient in the flesh. Ask these die-hards to turn their minds back to the dark days when they sat their qualification exams. How were they examined? Did they see patients – no! They saw photographs! Now there's a thought!

In this case, a telemedicine-based service is a better service and a better service inevitably means a bigger demand, so Health Authority finance directors look out! Of course it's not just the nurses who will become the 'David Baileys' and take the pictures – digital cameras only cost a few hundred pounds and if you buy the right computer you get one free.

Patients can take pictures too – don't forget that 10% of the population is brighter than doctors. Patients all over Manchester will be asking a close friend to snap their annoying little rash and email it off to the last remaining dermatologist in Europe, who lives in a luxury penthouse in Monte Carlo. We wouldn't be surprised if 'snap a rash' booths didn't start springing up in Tesco before long. The 'Derma King' (or Queen) will email a reply along with an electronic prescription, updating the GP along the way. Far fetched? The golden rule of technology is that if you can imagine it, it will probably happen.

And put some thought into the economics of the whole thing. The Derma King can charge half of what their now defunct traditional brethren used to charge and still clean up because he's cranking through five times as many in a given time. Five minutes a consult, 12 an hour at £30 a pop! Not bad, eh? The customers (GP or patient) are happy too because they have a fixed cost, and control over their destiny. No more 'See you in three months, Mrs Jones'.

Wait there's still more. We're on a roll

One of the very first teledermatology projects supported a nurse-led dermatology service on an island off the coast of Maine in the US. After a couple of years, the Docs on the mainland realised that they were no longer getting any consults and thought the kit must be broken or something. So they went over to see what the problem was. 'No problem', said the nurse, 'I know it all now'.

What had happened? She'd learnt on the job. Because she was receiving answers to questions the next morning (rather than the next year in Manchester), she was getting daily continuing medical education and if she wasn't sure, she had built up a nice archive she could refer back to.

<hr>

EXERCISE

Get the team together and take teledermatology as an example. Work through the changes that would have to take place to move from a traditional dermatology service to the brave new world.

Don't be shy. Perhaps dermatology will be better off outside of hospitals.

Don't forget the hard decisions. Positions may go. Clinics may change radically or disappear completely. Hospitals may lose funding. Dermatology may follow the dentists out of the NHS. What positive benefits might accrue from these apparently negative consequences?

EXERCISE

 Now go through the same process for your own project.

The key stages in change management

Again, no problem here. You've done most of the work. This section is all about looking at it from a different, or changing, perspective. Interesting stuff and worth the effort.

1 Define the scope of change that the TMed project will create – *how big is it?*

2 Diagnose the present situation – *where are you now?*

3 Create a vision of the desired future – *what does the future look like?*

4 Analyse the gap and manage the transition – *what's the difference between where you are now and where you want to be?*

5 Handle resistance – *who and what is going to make it tougher than it needs to be?*

6 Stabilise the new situation – *got there, now stay there!*

1   Define the scope of the project

Make a start by defining the scope of the TMed project. This seems so obvious that even experienced change masters forget to do it! By defining the scope at the outset you will minimise confusion, identify the likely consequences and prevent trouble brewing up for you later.

The purpose of the change must be identified, the scope of the project defined and the key players who may have the power to prevent the change, identified and involved.

Key questions to ask are:

• Is there an organisational problem that needs to be addressed by the TMed project – what is it?

• Are there defined parts of the organisation that need to change in order to address this problem?

• What are the benefits to be gained by undertaking this change – where are the wins?

• What are the consequences of doing nothing?

• Is there a price to change and is it worth paying?

You'll see that we've already satisfied ourselves regarding a lot of this stuff through the clinical and business case. What about doing nothing though?

2   What is the present situation?

You must get a clear picture of where you are starting from – the current situation in that part of the organisation undergoing the change. This process makes it easier to identify where the problems are likely to come from and what needs to be changed. This will help you to decide on where to focus to get a commitment to the change project.

This is the flip side of 'if it ain't broke, don't fix it'. This says 'treat what hurts'. There are various levels to look at and they all impact on one another and need to be looked at as interacting systems.

EXERCISE

 Level 1: Broad influences

- What are the broad trends in the environment that are causing the need for change?

(Think about Political, Economic, Social and Technological trends – what gurus call a PEST analysis.)

EXERCISE

 Level 2: Local 'stakeholder' demands

This looks at the other organisations with which your organisation is interacting and that will be impacted on by a TMed project.

- How healthy is your relationship with those who interact with you (e.g. secondary care, health authorities, social services, housing, voluntary sector etc)?

- Ask what do they expect from you, and what is the likely impact if you fail to meet their needs?

EXERCISE

 Level 3: Culture

An organisation's culture is sometimes described as 'the way things are done around here'.

A change of culture within the organisation, or within sub-sections of it, that is associated with a new TMed approach is a major, sometimes painful but often, necessary goal.

Are the organisation's norms in terms of vision, values and principles (another acronym 'VVP' – you'll be an expert yourself soon) at odds with the way things need to be done in the future?

EXERCISE

 Level 4: Core purpose

This is sometimes spelled out in a 'mission statement'.

- Does the organisation really know and understand its purpose?

- What services/functions are we currently delivering?

- What services/functions do we really need to be delivering?

EXERCISE

 Level 5: Internal design

Is the organisation designed in an effective way to deliver its objectives? How will TMed impact on these?

Things to look at here include tasks, people, structure, rewards, information and decision making.

EXERCISE

 Level 6: Service delivery

This level of diagnosis focuses on TMed change projects aimed at specific parts of an organisation, such as Clinical Directorates.

- Is the department fulfilling its planned activity levels and performance against expectations?

- Is it delivering this activity in a way that meets the needs of its 'consumers' and 'customers'? How will TMed change that?

- Are communication processes effective both within the department and with other parts of the organisation? How do you know?

- Are individuals within the department working together effectively? How do you measure it?

- Is there an overall sense of cohesiveness within the team? Does it 'feel good'?

3 Create a vision of the future you want

Buoyed up with the first flush of enthusiasm, it is easy to get a TMed enabled change project underway. Very often though they run out of steam because no one has any idea of what they are aiming for. This is the 'vision thing' and vision things are good. There are two famous quotes that apply here. The future guru, Alan Kay, said 'the best way to predict the future is to create it'. That's sort of in line with what we're doing here, right? The other guy who knows a thing or two about all this is Bezoid who said that 'visions and strategies linked to a clear sense of trends and scenarios make us better able to shape the future we prefer'. Who are we to disagree?

Change masters learn the trick of painting a picture of what the future looks like. Painting the picture helps secure commitment and enthusiasm and the whole team should be involved in painting the picture – what goes in it, what colour it is, what the textures are.

EXERCISE

 Here's an exercise to help you paint pictures. It's a team exercise that involves creative thinking.

- Ask each member of the group to think about their own ideal outcome for the TMed project. Give them 4 minutes thinking time.

- Ask each to share their ideas with the rest of the group. Have a facilitator, and use a flip chart, so everyone can see.

- Identify key similarities and differences.

- Create a shared vision of the future.

Write down here your team's thoughts about the future vision for your TMed project.

4 Analyse the gap and manage the transition

Once you have a clear picture of the current situation and the desired future, you have the starting and end point for your TMed project. Now you are ready for Stage 4: Identifying the gap between where you are and where you are going. We move now into managing the transition.

To establish the specific steps, undertake this 'gap analysis'. Go back to the previous exercises and look at what you need to do to finish the journey and arrive in your picture!

Objective review:

What needs to be done?	Objectives	By whom/By when?

 TIP

Make sure that someone is given, and accepts, overall responsibility for managing the change and ensuring that the plan is implemented. Someone has to 'wear the rose'. Oh, and make sure that they have the authority, resources and skills to do it.

Communication

Effective communication is critical to the success of any change management project, not least a TMed project, which is after all an exercise in communication, and one that is likely to be the focus of canteen gossip. Folk wondering if they will still have a job; if they are up to the project; if they have got the necessary skills; how it will impact on their daily life; if they will be more accountable; if it will be easier to measure their performance; and if they will be found wanting. Will they have a chance to shine, take on more responsibility, become a leader?

EXERCISE

   Write your own communication strategy.

We've all learned about 'spin' over the last few years. Mr Mandelson wouldn't call it that of course, he'd call it 'effective communication', but whatever you call it, it's important to get the right message across.

- What do we need to tell people? Usually everything, because if you don't tell, someone will.

- When are we going to tell them? The best advice is, 'as fast as you can'.

- Who is going to tell them? The best guide is 'the person with most authority' – this is not a good time to hide.

- How are we going to communicate? In person is always best – it's tough and takes time but pays its own reward. If not, there are always meetings, newsletters, email. People worried about change like to read what's going on in the messenger's eyes, not on a piece of paper.

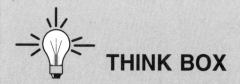 **THINK BOX**

Thanks to John's mate Brian for this one.

Brian is an excellent GP who is also top dog in his PCG and knows a thing or two about change. He is very concerned about NHS Direct and how it was introduced by our friends at the DoH. No consultation, no integration, a threat to GPs who are already providing a good service through the co-ops, all that sort of thing.

He's absolutely right of course, but . . .

Let's just assume, for the sake of argument, that NHS Direct is a good idea which will be the catalyst for transition to a single point of entry for out-of-hours calls which can quickly, efficiently and effectively manage all out-of-hours calls for the country. Major re-engineered change for the better – a blow for the good guys.

We know, we know. There's no evidence to back that up, but just accept that the politicians and the men from the ministry went over to the States, saw it in action in the health service there (6 million calls so far), saw the very positive results from a similar concept in banking, and really believe that it is a great idea. What are their options for getting it in?

How would you introduce a major innovative national service without becoming bogged down in interminable committees and endless debate? What process is in place to do that? How could it be done better?

Send us your answers in an email please because we don't know. If there isn't a good answer, do we as a community have a problem?

5 Handle resistance

People resist change for all sorts of reasons (*see* Step 8 on page 90). They are not very difficult to define and many of them can be anticipated. Planning to handle resistance is the change master's way of making sure resistance doesn't hold up the progress of your TMed project.

Here are some ways to get commitment to change and thereby reduce resistance:

- **Involvement** – make people feel part of what is going on

- **Visioning** – share the vision of the future, paint the picture

- **Communication** – tell 'em what's going on, remind 'em and tell 'em again!

- **'Treating what hurts'** – don't change for change's sake, do the bits that need doing

- **Knowing how individuals respond to change** – think about how you reacted to change, other people will feel the same way: unsure, cautious, worried, resentful, perhaps even relieved!

- **Encouraging people to develop new relationships** – take the best of the past into the future and emphasise the difference with new working partners.

6 Stabilise the new situation

Finally, the project needs to be evaluated, lessons need to be learned for future projects and the situation needs to be consolidated before embarking on any more change. Change piled upon change will cause discomfort and morale will take a dive.

Keep them up to speed with what is happening and let them see that it's making a difference.

What sort of incentives can you offer to make people feel good about the change?

EXERCISE

 Key questions to ask:

- What lessons have we learned from the TMed project?

- What worked well and what worked less well?

- What would you like to have done differently?

- Are there any development needs for individuals now that the project is up and running?

- What have I learnt about myself during this project?

Risk management for technophobes and sceptics

We know you are a big techie and a whizz at all this by now but we would be remiss if we didn't warn you about some of the few pitfalls and pratfalls you would do best to avoid.

Some 'dos' and 'don'ts':

- Do make sure that what you already have is Y2K compliant. If you don't know what Y2K means, try a career as a lamplighter or wick trimmer. (On the subject of Y2K, we've just seen a bulletin from the Microsoft Corporation saying that the release of Windows 2000 has been delayed. They are putting a brave face on it though and are confidant that it will be ready for the first quarter of 1901 – ho, ho!)

- Do think hard before you buy new kit. Don't forget about the procurement problems that the NHS has already got itself into. Where can you go to for advice? Can you trust the people who are selling you the stuff? Probably not – they want to sell it, don't they? Really good independent advice on IT is hard to come by. Beware! You have been warned.

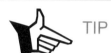 TIP

It's often not the technical specification of the software that lets you down, it's the hardware's operational memory – called RAM. Always go for the highest level of RAM you can afford and the most amount of conventional memory. Working systems eat memory, you'll be surprised how quickly it gets gobbled up.

- Do make sure you know what you want. Yes, we know it sounds banal to say it but look at it this way. Do you really need to buy the latest Pentium XYZ, with bells and whistles, or can you get a better deal by buying something with a less sexy specification? What do you really want the system to do?

- Do make sure you 'futureproof' the system. That means making sure it does not have redundancy built into it. Make sure it is upgradeable, flexible and will see you through well into the future.

- Do find out about the Data Protection Act – too big a subject to deal with here, so call them on 01625 545745. It's one of those annoying automated switchboard thingamajigs, but stick with it and you can get a very good leaflet, or the reward for being really determined is to get to speak to a human being.

- Keeping records on computer? Do something to ensure confidentiality. Don't leave screens full of data unattended, don't give your password to the practice receptionist or secretary or anybody (we know you do!). Who has access to patient records? If the price was right, who could have access to patient records? Think we're joking? How do you think private detectives get hold of the information they do? The answer is: easy money and sloppy people.

- Do make sure you back up your files. Don't worry too much about backing up system files – you can always reload the system. Do make sure you back up your data. There are all kinds of automated back up systems that will do it for you regularly.

- The best advice is.
    - back up data *every day*
    - critical stuff *twice a day*
    - and *one day* you'll be pleased you took this advice!

- Don't make it easy for your kit to be nicked. Do make sure you mark it all. The local police or crime prevention copper will be pleased to pay you a visit and help you get that sorted.

- Don't catch a virus. I don't mean one of those things that GPs say they can't do anything about. I mean a real virus that wipes out your computer. You can do something about them. First, be sure to install a virus checker. There are lots of systems that you can install. And don't forget to update them every three months at least. Suppliers will do it free for the first year or so and a good one only costs £40 anyway. Try looking at www.drsolomon.com No access to the web? Go and get it, now! Come to regard computer viruses as the digital equivalent of HIV rather than the common cold, and you won't go too far wrong.

- Do fit a surge protector for your PCs. What's a surge protector? Well, PCs can be sensitive to the amount of electricity going through them. The UK system works between 220 and 240 volts. Although the PC reduces the voltage to something much smaller, it can be sensitive to a surge (or spike) in the supply. Nasty spikes mean blank screens and misery. PC shops and DIY stores sell extension sockets that have surge protectors and smooth out the spikes. Only a few quid and well worth the investment. You can also get a smart socket that stores up just enough juice for you to shut your system down with dignity and style if the electricity supply fails. They're called UPSs (Uninterruptable Power Supplies) and are available for the price of a large G&T with ice and a slice – money well spent.

- Don't allow games on your PCs. They can encourage the computer nervous to have fun and get to grips with the machine – we guess there is an argument for that. But they take up space and are best taken off. However, don't under any circumstances allow anyone to load their own games – why should they be playing games in your time and who knows what nasty viruses they might deposit on your hard disk?

What about email?

If you agree that the NHS is very good at getting itself into a mess over IT, computers and technology, believe us, you ain't seen nothin' yet! There is another disaster waiting just around the corner. The millennium bug is a flea bite by comparison. The message is – it is the messages that will cause the problem.

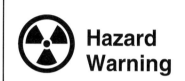 **Hazard Warning**

If experiences in the private sector are anything to go by, the NHS has no idea what it is letting itself in for with email.

Patient appointments, pathology results, internal messaging, ordering and countless other tasks are set to become electronic. All GPs will be hooked up with email, as will most managers and hospital consultants.

Litigation, writs and battles are just an email away. The problems will start internally and then the outside world will come crashing down on the heads of an unsuspecting NHS management.

The potential for problems identified itself in the US last March. It was reported that the merchant bankers Morgan Stanley and Dean Witter & Co, agreed an out-of-court settlement with two of its employees. Reason? Some member of staff had circulated a bad taste joke about Afro-Americans on the internal email system. The aggrieved staff reached for their lawyers and the company reached for its cheque book. The court was about to decide that employers are responsible for all internal email traffic, regardless of its origination. Morgan Stanley apparently settled. This is just part of what the NHS can expect. Other lawsuits alleging everything from sexual discrimination to breach of confidence, have been sparked by companies without proper email policies and planning.

Industry has been caught unprepared by the impact of email. A Gallup Poll, conducted in the US in May 99, found that the typical office worker in a decent sized corporation would deal with up to 60 incoming and outgoing emails in a day. There are about 156 000 administrative and estates staff in the NHS (to say nothing of the doctors and nurses). That could mean, when they all get the hang of email, potential for nine million messages whizzing around the system every day. Controlling the content of all the messages is an impossible job.

Should a PCG, Trust, GP or any other health employer become involved in a court case or industrial tribunal, electronic mail is ready to provide some more shocks. A legal device, known as 'discovery', can be used to force litigants to reveal every file, note and piece of

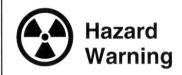 **Hazard Warning**

Planting a blank email into a file history makes it possible, at a later stage, to go back and fill it in with any message you like. A trick likely to fool everyone, even an experienced observer.

paper they have that might be pertinent to the case in question. Nothing may be hidden. Courts can prise open your filing cabinets and archives. They can plug into your hard disk too. If the records they want to see include email messages that have been deliberately erased or modified, you could find yourself up in front of the beak for contempt of court.

Industry is spending millions setting up record management systems, policies and organisational structures to manage the invisible tide of email.

The simple answer? Treat electronic messages like paper messages and file them – the gurus call it 'e-archiving'. Unfortunately, this is not so simple. Deciding what to keep and what to dump becomes a major problem. What to retain and for how long is a policy decision and you must have a proper written policy about it, approved by the Board of whatever comfy corner of the NHS you live in. Get it right as you may have to answer for it in court or in front of the Public Accounts Committee.

Emails can easily be faked or fiddled with and printed out messages can be similarly counterfeited. A storage system that is tamperproof does not come cheap and will eat up a storage disk faster than an American termite can chomp its way through a house.

So-called e-shredding software exists and is one way of zapping messages that could come back to haunt you. However, hidden history and cache files in Windows and other systems can leave a trail of clues that the determined, computer literate can follow. Emptying the 'Re-cycle bin' does not mean 'gone for good'. Any spook worth his or her salt can retrieve stuff you erased months ago, even though you can't retrieve things you lost when one of those annoying little 'Are you sure' windows came up and you clicked the wrong box.

Email will become fundamental to the way the NHS runs its affairs. The service needs some rules and guidance – fast.

Here are six ideas to avoid e-fail with email:

Check

1   Warn all staff with an 'on-screen' message about the practice's rules for email.

2   Make it clear that email is not confidential and will be routinely monitored. More importantly, hammer home the fact that email is not a substitute for the kind of conversation that used to take place in the canteen, lavatory or lift.

3   Stamp out digital gossip, bar the transmission of personal mail, jokes, smutty material and non-business messages. American experience shows that offended staff can sue their employer – someone is bound to try a case here, sooner or later.

4   Set up in-house e-training to help staff understand the rules. This might persuade a court that you have taken your responsibilities seriously. Incorporate email policies into contracts of employment.

5   Install one of the new programmes to monitor email for key words and phrases, to flag up offensive material and tell everyone you've done it.

6   Decide on archive policies now. What to keep, how long to keep it, how to keep it and who is responsible. Cost electronic archive processes and budget for it – the outlay is more than you think. Disk and tape space doesn't come cheap – but not as expensive as a few days at the High Court!

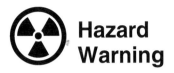 **Hazard Warning**

Never, never, never open an attachment to an email that has the suffix EXE. Unless it came from your Mother and even then be suspicious. These types of files are a favourite vehicle for the lunatics who spread viruses. We keep banging on about viruses but they really are a major pain in the backside, they're very common and they will make your life a complete misery if you get one. This is another 'if you do nothing else after reading this book' message, so pay attention.

Come to think about it don't open any attachment to an e-message if you have no idea who the sender is. These days the lunatics can infect your machine with word processing files and all manner of other stuff.

So, there you have it. Send off for the MBA and let's get back to the main business of getting the thing implemented.

Now on to the last three steps . . .

Step 10: Phased implementation

A quick revision of the principles we learned when we looked at the clinical and business case. The implementation plan will need to be written for those who will be doing the implementing. Who are they?

Is the plan for:

- People in your department to give them a sense of direction and clarity?

- Your boss or a group of people who have the power to say 'yes' or 'no'?

- People who will 'invest' or fund the project or service?

- People who will use the service?

- People who will work in the service and run it?

- People who will give permission for the project to get underway?

- . . . perhaps it will be a combination of all of them.

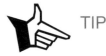 TIP

When you produce the plan put yourself in the shoes of the person who will read it and make the decisions to enable it to happen. Be honest with yourself. Does it make sense and can you deliver?

 TOP TIP

What will they need to get out of the plan to help them make a decision? Write your plan through the readers' eyes.

The implementation plan

The implementation phase is where the rubber meets the road. The same principles hold for this bit as they did for the planning phase, except that real money will be involved now and mistakes will cost. You've made your decision to go for it, now you have to deliver. If the implementation is a cock up, the whole project is at risk.

Planning, as ever, is the key.

The plan must answer at least four questions:

1 What is your activity now?

2 Are you competing for approval or resources? If so, how are you different (what makes you the best choice?) *or* can you demonstrate you have satisfied the key requirements for approval?

3 What are your tactics, what do you need to do to win approval or resources to turn your plan into reality?

4 What are the benefits? Such as improvement in health gain or greater efficiency.

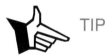 TIP

It is unlikely you will have all the information you need at your fingertips, in order to complete the plan.

- Whose support do you need to complete the plan?
- Who do you need to talk to to gather the information that is required?
- Who are the other stakeholders?
- What does it mean in terms of their time and yours?

Matching diaries is never easy when folk are busy. Is your timescale realistic?

What goes into the plan? Here's a quick overview:

1 The name of the organisation writing the plan

Is the plan for a department or project where the name is different or new? Think about how the name is to be selected?

- Will there be a competition?
- Will the name be based on geography, a focal point in the area?
- Will the name conflict with one that is already in use?

- Is the name credible and will it stand the test of time?

- Does the name identify what you do?

- Is the name an ego trip for the organisation or will it mean something to the public?

- Make sure the acronym isn't something rude (remember the Forward Advanced Resuscitation Teams).

EXERCISE

Describe how the name of the project might be chosen. If the name has already been chosen, is there 'buy in' to the name? Do people like it, do they identify with it? Does it matter? Think about the plan you are about to write and ask if there is a title or a short phrase that would crystallise its purpose. Write it here:

2 Does the project have a home?

At this stage the project will develop beyond the corner of a desk.

EXERCISE

- Is the project to be housed in appropriate accommodation?

- Is there a need to take into account the possibility of growth and a new home? What are the timescales?

- What are the practicalities of finding a new home?

- Are offices available?

- Does planning consent have to be sought?

- What does that mean in terms of time?

- What about telephone lines, kit, stationery and all that boring stuff?

3 Does the organisation have a mission statement to help focus everyone on the same goals?

Organisations are never what they seem. A delivery company does not just deliver parcels – they deliver our goods in one piece, on time and without delay. A restaurant is not a restaurant – it is a quick snack, a romantic evening or a business lunch.

> Write your mission statement here (for those who didn't flick straight to here, it's on the notice board – for those who did, there's more stuff about this in Step 1).

4 Who is going to be responsible for writing the plan?

Organising the detail of the implementation plan, collating the information and drafting takes time. Who is going to do it? Do they have a day job and are they trying to fit this project in with everything else in their in-tray? Is it practical? Is the research phase resourced?

Consider what new people you will need to run and develop your project or plan, and allow lead time for recruiting, induction and training. Lead times for senior managers can run to 2–3 months.

 TIP

Very few people really do hit the ground running. If you need to hire staff, remember that anyone who is any good will already be doing a good job for someone else; allow time for them to disengage from their current employment and allow time for induction and settling in.

EXERCISE

- What extra skills does the organisation need?

- Are there sufficient skills in the organisation?

- Is extra training required?

- Do people have the time to deliver?

- Are you dumping responsibilities on willing shoulders that will eventually fail?

5 Time for some more finance stuff – sorry!

Not all plans need to have detailed financial information in them. Most do, but not all. The type of plan that does not need financial detail might be an introductory document designed for internal use that clarifies issues such as structure and who does what.

However, most plans will need some financial data to back them up. Here are the main headings that financial details will fall under:

A balance sheet: This is an overall position statement setting out the value of the organisation, its assets, income and expenditure.

A profit and loss account: Not in the NHS, surely? 'Profit and loss' is an expression commonly used in the business community and hardly needs a definition. In the NHS, where profits are not made, it is probably easier to think of it as income and expenditure. Think of it as managing surpluses or losses on activity, manpower and finances.

A cash flow forecast: Cash flow is seen as the lifeblood of most business. Companies that trade at the margins of profitability can sometimes keep going, for longer than they should, because they have a positive, regular and healthy cash flow. It is also true that very profitable organisations have crashed because cash flow has been poor and they have run out of money.

The public sector is fortunate in that it has a 'draw-down' arrangement with the Treasury and cash flow is not such an issue. The flow of cash through the organisation is a concern for directors of finance who need to know when they are likely to be called upon to make payments, and when they are to expect receipts.

All this gets turned on its head if there is an unexpected demand on services, such as in the winter months, and there is not enough cash in the system to pay the bills. That's why the Gods of Whitehall come up with money for the 'winter crisis'.

Is your plan vulnerable to a finance director who has to give unexpected financial priority to some other part of the organisation? How sure are you of the availability of the resources you will need to get going? Probably worth popping around to the finance director for a cup of coffee and a reality check if you're not sure.

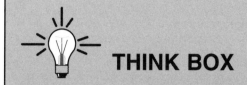

THINK BOX

Health is increasingly encouraged to work creatively with partners outside the NHS – organisations such as social services and some others in the private and voluntary sector. If a project is to be joint funded or to come from the newly 'pooled budget' arrangements with social services, think about timescales.

The public sector financial year runs April to March. Is that the same for everyone you are involved with? Are different accounting arrangements within different organisations likely to be a problem?

Keeping up to date with what is happening

Make sure your plan allows for regular up date of the financial situation. Don't be shy about circulating budgets to the team. People have got to know where they are – good or bad.

Regular reports are called 'management accounts'. They should be produced regularly and consistently, in the same format (preferably graphically), so that it is easy to identify trends. They must be detailed enough to be interesting and helpful, but simple enough to be clear.

IT buffs should be able to find an accounting package that is capable of displaying complex information in graphical and simple-to-understand ways.

Software is cheap and misunderstandings expensive. Graphs, bar charts and graphics can compare last month with this month and the year to date with targets – easy!

EXERCISE

 How financially literate are the people you work with? It's OK not to be an accountant! Honest! The important thing is that reports are regular and everyone who has responsibility understands what's going on.

Develop a system for financial reporting that is accurate and comprehensive enough so you don't get caught out, but responsive enough so you can get things done.

- Who will hold and be responsible for the budget?

- What does technology have to offer?

- What are the checks and balances?

- Who can authorise expenditure and at what levels?

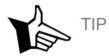

TIP

It is a good plan to get the finance director involved here. There is likely to be a spotlight on your project and it is best that someone else has the headache and responsibility for the cash. The chain to the cheque needs to be short and you need to try to establish a fast track system and avoid going to committees or through tiers of bureaucracy to get things done.

Most finance directors are good folk who will help where they can. Your project will probably be fairly high profile if you've got the communication bit right, in which case the finance director may ask one of his team to keep a watchful eye over you (if so, make sure you include them and make them feel a part of your team too).

Start up projects, using pump-priming funds, are the sort that will require a business case and may legitimately not have their income matching their expenditure. The shortfall may be picked up elsewhere. Be careful to make realistic projections and if there is an excess of expenditure over income, don't hide it. The key is to be realistic.

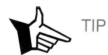

TIP

Be sure to be realistic with projections and if there is an excess of expenditure over income, don't hide it. The key is to be realistic.

Decide over what period you can realistically forecast in detail. In the world of business, high volume, high turnover activity is measured in weeks and months. Low volume, low turnover in months and years.

Think of a forecast as a photograph of how you see activity taking place. A careful picture of the detail up close and a snap of what the view might be from further away.

6 Phasing

How do you eat an elephant? Answer: elephant kebabs, elephant steak, elephant burgers, elephant stew.

Get the message? Bit by bit.

That's the whole point of phasing. If you try and implement in a big bang, all you'll get is a loud noise, a lot of deaf colleagues and a mess on the carpet. Remember, success by an inch is a synch. Success by a yard is hard.

You haven't come all this way to do a pilot project either. Pilots are for the feint hearted who haven't done their planning properly or who are trying some whizz bang new technology for the first time. They have fixed end points, accept the possibility of failure and they are not allowed as readers of this book.

EXERCISE

   Devise a phasing programme for a district wide store and forward dermatology project. There are 250 practices in the area, four Trusts and three dermatologists.

Now look at your project and break it down into bite-sized chunks.

---

7   Write the technical implementation plan

This is where you can get your techie out of his box again. This is his job but it is essential that the technical plan is integrated with the financial plan, and with the wider implementation plan. You also need to make sure that your phasing plan makes technical sense. Make sure, especially, that the kit is installed at roughly the same time the training programme kicks in. (Oh, we know it might be obvious, but we could tell you a story or two about folk being trained with no kit and vice versa.)

EXERCISE

 Who should be in your implementation team? It will probably be based on the original planning team but there may well be a few changes, and a few more folk will certainly become involved as things hot up.

Get the team together and work out an integrated implementation plan to include:

- The sensible sequence of events

- The show stoppers

- The process to review progress towards implementation

TIP

In Progress Reviews (IPRs)

Good idea, these. They are simply regular roundtable meetings where everyone turns up to report on progress. If they are linked to a task list and a project timeline, they provide a powerful incentive to perform.

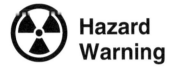 **Hazard Warning**

Vapour ware

This is the technical world's very own version of bulls**t and anyone with any experience of techies will know what we mean. There is always some 'latest version' coming out which will be much 'better, faster and cheaper' than what is available now. But the specification is not available till next week and we won't know the price until at least three weeks on Monday. Beware. Never happens.

- Give them your requirement
- Give them your service levels
- Give them a realistic date when you expect to have the money and be ready to put it in.

And set a date for the presentation of the results – in pen!

9 Key decision dates

Think through all the stages that will take you to the first day of the operation of your plan (or new service). Buying equipment, finding premises, recruiting staff and the host of little tasks that make for a complete and done job.

Sometimes it is easier to work back from a known starting date. The 'work back' approach is very useful, particularly when it reveals that to get to where you want to be in three months time, you should have started four weeks ago!

EXERCISE

Develop a schedule of key decision dates working back from the end point, and make some realistic decisions about timescales.

TOP TIP

Have you noticed that on the wing mirrors of some cars there are etched the words 'Objects in this mirror may be closer than they appear'? Try a similar tack with your project calendar and diary (and your techie's):

'The dates in this project plan may be closer than they appear'

Tempus fugit when you're having fun.

10 Buying some kit?

If your plan envisages the acquisition of any capital equipment, you must detail what it is, and how its purchase is to be financed.

EXERCISE

 List all the capital items (costing more than £300) required in the first three years, including (in each case) how it will be purchased – lease, loan, cash, rent etc.

Capital item	Inital cost	Time of anticipated purchase	Method of payment	Completion of loan etc

Plus:

- What is the procurement process for new items? Are items to be researched and selected or is a specification to be drawn up and bids invited? Who is going to do it and by when?

- Where is the line of accountability?

- Draw up a complete list of the equipment you will need to get you started. Consider how they will be financed.

What are the procurement issues?

When the history of the NHS comes to be written, it will be the graveyard stories of how the NHS screwed up IT procurement that will occupy the headlines. Whilst the world tooled itself up to the eyeballs, the NHS was left blushing.

Why? Simple answer, the NHS wasn't sure what it wanted to buy and didn't get what it wanted.

As a publicly accountable organisation there are rules you must follow.

 First stop is a cup of coffee with the finance director. He will introduce you to the dark arts of standing financial instructions (SFIs). These are very boring sets of documents that will explain how finances, including procurement, is supposed to be done.

Tell your new finance friend how much you want to spend. There will be a set of 'threshold limits'. This is finance speak that means up to a certain level you can spend taxpayers' money with a particular person's authority. After that level someone else has to do it, and so on. There will be a set of limits that take you up to the prospect of needing God's signature and authority.

The SFIs will also set out how you buy things. Again, they work on a set of limits. Up to a certain amount you can probably pop into Woolworths on the way home and pick one up. At the next level, the organisation may have gone through a process to determine a regular supplier. After that you will probably have to invite tenders. It all depends on how much you want to spend. There is also the added complication of European stuff – groan, too much to deal with in detail here. Suffice to say that after a certain threshold you have to advertise the tenders across Europe in a magazine called the *European Journal*, otherwise known as the EJ.

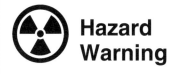 **Hazard Warning**

We know what you are thinking – *no*! You can't simply break a big contract down into a little one just to avoid the threshold rules. If you do, you'll go to jail.

Here is a procurement checklist to help you keep out of jail!

Got it!

1 All public procurement is based on propriety, regularity and value for money.

2 Value for money is the optimum combination of whole life cost/quality and fitness for purpose. (So, you don't always have to pick the cheapest.)

3 Public procurement must be in line with EU requirements.

4 The purpose of procurement is to meet the users' requirements – state them clearly. You must know what you want. Take time to be sure.

5 Goods and services must be acquired by competition appropriate to the value and complexity of what is required.

6 Market testing is the only way to ensure value for money.

7 Dealings with suppliers and potential suppliers must be based on honesty, integrity, impartiality and objectivity.

8 Selection criteria for prospective bidders must be transparent, open and not necessarily based on size.

9 Award criteria must be spelled out.

10 Evaluation of bids should involve appropriate techniques for assessing value for money.

11 Public bodies are required to pay their suppliers on time. Where there is no other agreement, 30 days from the date of receipt of valid invoice.

12 Purchasers can agree any terms of the contracts they enter into except variation in price, which should not extend beyond two years, and prompt payment clauses.

13 Purchasers cannot enter into contracts with other parts of the same legal entity – but you can enter into service level agreements.

14   You can use a purchasing agency to act on your behalf, such as NHS Supplies, the Buying Agency, CCTA and the Government Purchasing Agency, Northern Ireland.

15   Private sector agents may be used provided they comply with all the rules that would have applied to you if you had done the job yourself.

So now you know!

The golden rules on procurement:

- Be clear about what you want.
- Be clear what represents value for money.
- Stick to the procurement rules.
- Make sure you got what you wanted.

EXERCISE

 Define a procurement strategy for a teleconferencing link between three centres (in three trusts).

Assume you have complied with procurement rules and concentrate on what constitutes value for money.

But also note that you not only have VTC boxes to procure, but also communication links and call charges on into the future. Consider the advantages and disadvantages of a prime contractor concept where one company has a consortium behind it *versus* you dealing with a number of different contractors yourself.

Who can help?

Procurement, step by step:

- Establish the threshold rules.

- Define the kit you want – be sure about the specification, and include support and back up requirements.

- Does it constitute value for money?

- Market test.

- Agree terms of payment.

- Let contract.

- Did you get what you want?

This is important stuff.

Be sure to define the new work process:

So you think you can make a go of it? Good! But look out! This is going to mean changes in the way the service is run and the way people work. The new work processes need to be identified and agreed with staff. Scheduling and clinics may need to be altered and some provision may need to be made for totally new concepts such as specialists working from home. How are you going to manage and communicate the change to your customers – patients, GPs, whoever?

There may also be a change in the balance of work. For example, many telemedicine services will enable patients

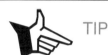 TIP

Don't forget to make the necessary changes to job descriptions and contracts of employment. These days you can only do it with consent. If in doubt, get advice. Who from? The head honcho of either the local Human Resources Department or NHS Trust should be able to tell you.

to remain at home or in the primary care setting, so that hospital infrastructure costs will fall, whereas those in primary care will rise. Specialist time taken on an episode of care may also change – substantially lower with store and forward consultations and probably somewhat longer using video teleconferencing. The organisations using the telemedicine service will need to address these issues and modify their current arrangements to allow for them.

You will need the team to help out with this one but you will also have to be at your most sensitive. This will be crunch time for a lot of folk, their expectations, dreams or fears will almost certainly not be the same as your plans. What is greater efficiency to you is less hours or no job for others.

Be gentle, be consistent, be straight. Use your middle tier people to help make sure that the new work process makes sense, and perhaps go through a few paper exercises or walk throughs to test them. They are also a great asset to reinforce what is happening and to back check that expectations are at least in the right ballpark.

EXERCISE

Document your new re-engineered work practice. Does it make sense?

Don't forget that TMed by definition has at least two ends which are probably in different organisations. What is the plan to make sure that your new work processes fit in with theirs? Think about an arbitration mechanism should you disagree.

Quick check

Have you . . .

Got the process sorted out? Who will have overall responsibility for finalising the plan? If members of the team are contributing individual segments of the plan, is there a timetable for them to work to? Who is doing the checking, reminding and collating?

What about the people?

The project will almost certainly have some impact on all or most of your team and the team at the other end of the link. Do you need more staff or less? Some people may need to move on, others promoted.

EXERCISE

 Write out your current team structure and who is where. Then write out the team as it will be once you're up and running.

- Work out who will move where.

- Who will need additional training.

- Work out your short-term and longer-term plan to move from your current to the future manning structure.

- Will anyone lose their job, and how will you handle it?

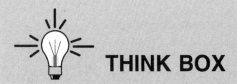

THINK BOX

Change can be good. It can be a good time to make changes that might otherwise have been too difficult. Are there other underlying structural changes in your organisation that you can slip through under cover of a telemedicine project?

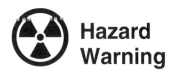

Hazard Warning

Do not underestimate the impact of even small changes that a TMed project can bring about in an organisation.

Decided on the format of the plan's presentation? Think about style. How do you plan to do the . . .

Headings

And what is the length of the body copy? Keep it simple, avoid technical language and use:

- bullet points
- to emphasise
- important points.

Steer clear of **fancy** typefaces as they are a pest to read. Use Times Roman for the text and Arial for the headings and leave the fancy stuff to the designers of perfume packaging.

Plan the pages. You should aim for something like this:

Front page (cover) – nothing fancy, the more businesslike the better, avoid scans, pictures, clip art and cartoons. If you are using colour, use black for all the text and use colour sparingly. Except for graphs, don't use more than one other colour.

Contents page for easy reference – not everyone who sees your plan will want to read all of it. Make sure the contents page is comprehensive and accurate.

Mission statement – reproduce your mission statement and let readers see where you are coming from and show you've thought about it.

Introduction to the organisation – a brief pen portrait of the project, its location, the number of staff and so on. Try and give people a feel for the organisation.

Objectives in publishing the plan – this is a detailed section on what the project intends to do and why.

Action plan – stating how you intend to achieve your objectives and the deadlines you intend to keep to.

Detailed supporting information – such as financial statements and projections and technical documents.

 ## On target? How good is your plan?

Seven steps to evaluate the plan:

1   Is it realistic? Can the project meet its financial obligations and formation criteria?

2   Where capital developments are involved, is there enough money in the system to pay for them and keep them running?

3   Does the plan fit in with national guidelines and local healthcare target imperatives (*Health of The Nation* and HImPs)? You do not exist in a vacuum. Indeed health is increasingly set to play a role alongside other agencies in addressing disease.

4   Does it demonstrate complete control over all resources? Nothing left to chance and estimates (where absolutely necessary) based on conservative thinking?

5   Where applicable, thoroughly thought through strategies to deal with investment.

6   If any reliance is placed on non-NHS income (grants for staff or development from pharmaceutical companies, for example), what happens when the financing ends?

7   What is the sensitivity of the key assumptions, particularly around staff competencies? Are they realistic?

Phew! We bet you're pleased to get that lot out of the way!

   Time for a cup of coffee – or something stronger!

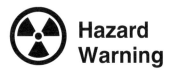 **Hazard Warning**

This is a break point and is the third 'go/no go' decision.

Step 11: Training, training, training and more training

You've heard it all before: 'Training is essential', 'We should have paid more attention to training' and so on. But it's always the first thing to go when the budget gets tight and no-one ever really does it properly, at least not in the NHS. Well, it just doesn't seem fun – back to school, boring lectures, we're far too busy doing actual work.

Well, it just won't do! This has got to be done right. After all this effort this is your last chance to grasp defeat from the jaws of victory. Training really is essential and you really do need to pay a lot of attention to it, although not in the way that immediately springs to mind.

Using the kit

Staff ain't daft. With a bit of encouragement they can work wonders. They don't leave their brains behind when they come to work – we just treat them like they do! When they're on holiday or at a family gathering, most folk can take a picture. Heaven knows how many sit in front of a computer pressing the right keys. And besides, you've spent a lot of time and effort making sure that the kit is really easy to use, so this part of the training should be easy.

Well it is but it still needs to be done, so . . .

EXERCISE

 Devise a method for assessing the present skills of staff who will be involved in an IT project using digital cameras and PCs.

Find a way of evaluating the outcomes and developing a training programme. Make it fun, relevant and hands on. Where possible, train folk to use the kit in the place they'll actually be using it – what the gurus call 'situational training'. (Another phrase for you to show off with!)

Training should obviously reflect what you want to achieve. It's about giving your team the necessary skills, insight and understanding to really want to do business the new way. The technology is easy (see every chapter so far in this book), it's the re-engineering that's difficult and that's where you need to focus the major part of your training efforts.

You'll have done a lot of it already. The team has been involved in working out the re-engineered solution and so it should make sense and be workable. You've also included them at each step along the way, and they'll have as much invested in this as you. The cards are stacked well in your favour.

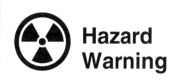

Hazard Warning

. . . technology is easy, it's the re-engineering that's difficult and that's where you need to focus the major part of your training efforts.

But this is big change and it has to work right on day one, otherwise people will begin to question the whole idea and the 'neah sayers' will start to emerge from the dark recesses of your department.

As you start to devise your training programme, bear in mind the following principle:

'Train as you fight, fight as you train.'

Another lesson from the military who spend most of their time training and seem to be pretty good at it. It means realistic training, done by and large under the same conditions that you'll do the real thing in. It also means hands on, practical training not boring lectures.

Timing

Obviously the logical extension to this is that they should train on the kit they're going to use. This means some co-ordination on your part because you will be keen to get the project moving once you've got the kit, but on the other hand you can't until they're properly trained.

Work to training objectives

Break down the process into its constituent parts and define the standard that you will accept for each. Achieving those standards become your training objectives.

Introduce, educate, consolidate

This means you don't just do it once. Introduce a new concept ahead of time and train it in detail. And, once you're happy they've understood it, move on. And then come back to it and consolidate what you've trained some time later.

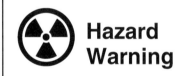 **Hazard Warning**

Training is an art in itself and not everyone is good at it, so choose well and establish a mechanism to assess the trainers. A side-effect of this approach is that you develop a natural troubleshooting hierarchy within your organisation that can deal with most problems as they arise.

Bite-sized chunks

Train in easy-to-digest steps and then join them up together into a whole. Once they've got the hang of that, start bowling occasional 'googlies' and gradually speed things up until they feel confident and know they're good – and, most important, know that day one of the real thing will be a piece of cake.

Train the trainers

If yours is a big project it can be logistically difficult and expensive to train everyone centrally. One answer is to train a group of trainers within your organisation who will go round and train the rest.

If you do this, it is important to remember that you have to train them in 'how' to train, as well as 'what' to train.

Tests

We may be a bit reactionary when we suggest 'tests'. We don't care! It works. Give 'em a test and make the test important. It concentrates the mind, gives them a challenge and a sense of achievement when they pass. Make it perfectly clear that the test will be based purely on the training objectives and will be, as far as possible, practical and based on their real world.

Reward success

Use your word processing skills and make up some certificates. Get the boss down to present them and make a fuss of the qualifiers.

This is to

Certify

_____

(Name)

_____

(Department)

Has successfully completed

_____

(Insert here the level achieved: phase 1, introductory, keyboard, full or whatever)

Training Course

at

_____

(Name of organisation)

Telemedicine Project

Date   Signed

By the way, we don't mind if you scan this in and use it!

Total bulls**t? No, it makes a difference! Take the rewarding of achievement seriously.

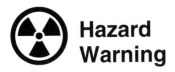 **Hazard Warning**

Remember if they get 80% in the test, they don't know 20% of what you've decided is important. Take the results personally. They're a reflection on you too.

EXERCISE

- Devise a set of training objectives for your project.

- Determine who will co-ordinate the training and who will train what.

- Write out your training plan.

- Work out how you will evaluate success.

Step 12: Evaluation

Truth time! How was it for you? Was it any good? How do you know? If your little heart has been set on a TMed project and you've put everything you've got into it – who is gonna tell you it ain't no good? The best judge is you. Can you do it? Have you got the intestinal fortitude!

But quite apart from the natural curiosity of an enquiring mind and the pride you get from knowing that at least you think it was worth it, there are a couple of even better reasons for evaluation.

First:

If you don't measure it, you can't make it better.

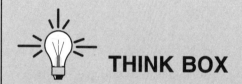

THINK BOX

True isn't it? That's what audit is all about. Do you feel better about audit now?

Early insight into evolving problems – this rings a bell

Americans never make mistakes, they have opportunities to improve. It's an entirely different mindset and the early insight idea comes out of the same mould.

If you have an evaluation process in place as you go along, then you'll spot the clangers when they're only tinkles, and you can then take steps to head them off at the pass.

It has to be said that one of the best barometers of how things are going is the staff. They know the score and you need to make sure there is a big wide road from them direct to you. If the messages stop arriving and it all goes quiet and they stop moaning, then you are probably way down the slippery slope.

Money

It's not your money that you're spending and you owe it to the taxpayer to make sure you spend it wisely. 'I'm a taxpayer so it is my money', we hear you cry. Not good enough.

They will let you have the money for the proof of concept phase of your project and only give you the rest when you can prove that it's money well spent, and you've achieved the target you set yourself (so make sure you set them carefully).

Defeating the forces of darkness and inertia

The NHS is dreadful at passing on good news. There's no mechanism for passing a really good idea from one place to the next and so the forces of darkness and inertia win by default.

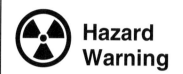 **Hazard Warning**

The NHS is dreadful at passing on good news. There's no mechanism for passing a really good idea from one place to the next and so the forces of darkness and inertia win by default.

You 'get up and go' types can't have that. So publish. Get people to invite you to nice places to talk about what you've done – start a web site (if Roy can do it you can – he gets 3000 visitors to his site each week from folk all over the globe). Do whatever you want but tell people what a wonderful thing you've done and show them the figures to back it up. Put some science behind what is still at the Basil Fawlty School of Evidence-Based Medicine. We all know it works but the sceptics want proof.

Again, you've done all the work. The matrices are all there, so please at the very least, give us a good quality outcome study to further the cause.

How to do it

As we've just mentioned, evaluation should be a piece of cake. It's basically the business case – but ongoing. All your variables are there complete with your starting position and where you are going to end up over a defined period of time.

EXERCISE

So just take a few minutes, it shouldn't take much longer, and pull out the business case. Write down the things that were important for you to improve on the left-hand side of a page with your starting figures next to them. Then decide on how often it makes sense to reassess them, bearing in mind which of the reasons for doing it, listed above, flicked your switch.

Who are you going to get to collect all the data? Being an entrepreneur type, you may well not be ideal. Besides, you're going to be way too busy.

Write it up and send it to the *BMJ, Health Service Journal, The British Journal of Healthcare Computing, Healthcare Today, Doctor Magazine, Hospital Doctor, Lancet, The News of the World* – anywhere, just get it published.

Section 6

Telemedicine in practice

One of the consequences of the war in Kosovo, among other horrors, was the residue of anti-personnel mines and cluster bombs that took a dreadful and unpublicised toll of the civilian population returning to their homes. The British Army provided medical support for the military personnel, as well as some very badly injured civilians.

What follows are some extracts from the email traffic that accompanied digital photographs, data, scans, X-rays and advice that was part of the telemedicine support. Read it and tell us that TMed can't change things.

I just got back from Kosovo. Great visit. Our folks are really doing a good job. Spent some time with the Brits in Pristina. They gave us a 'telemedicine' demonstration. Here's what they are doing. They have a digital camera, a tripod, a laptop computer and a printer. Total equipment cost of about $5000. They take pictures of X-rays on the light box, download the digital image to the laptop, and email it to wherever they want to send it via the Internet. They also take pictures with the digital camera of wounds and surgical procedures that are forwarded in the same manner. Pictures are also used for in-house training purposes. That's it. That's what they are doing. They have no motion capability, not even VTC. They are happy and satisfied with this very inexpensive and relatively unsophisticated set-up. That's my report. Hope you and the family are well. Talk to you later.

Here's another – note the last few words.

> A quick update, written at 0715 hrs, Thursday 15 July – yesterday afternoon, after I sent ***** (and you) the photos and details of the abdo-fistulae patient in Pristina ITU, I rang ***** to discuss the patient with him because of my need to get a second opinion asap. ***** worked for years as senior lecturer with Prof ***** at the *****, specialising in the management of Crohn's and complex fistula surgery, and I had worked as senior registrar for some two months on his unit. ***** is now a senior consultant there. He advised laparotomy asap, a proximal defunctioning jejunostomy, resection of any dubious/leaking/fistulous bowel, irrigation and leaving the abdo open as a laparostomy.
>
> The jejunostomy would effectively cause temporary intestinal failure, so he would need TPN for some time while healing proceeded. As we do not have TPN at our field hospital, that clarifies the options open to us – he either gets this type of treatment at Pristina, or needs transfer elsewhere. I am off in a few minutes to meet ***** (who coincidentally used to work with ***** as registrar! and they know each other well) and to see the patient for the first time.
>
> I was able to appreciate the patient's condition by looking at the photos taken by my ortho colleague yesterday – it really did help me to understand the situation and clarify my discussion with ***** – all before I have even met the patient. Telemedicine – it changes your practise.

Still not convinced? Try this.

> Many thanks for your excellent and very prompt advice re this unfortunate patient. I received the emails whilst discussing the case here with a Lebanese GI surgeon (who works for the Greek branch of Medicins du Monde), who will be operating with me tomorrow in Pristina hospital. I shall update you thereafter. The text files transmitted perfectly and are a real boon.
>
> Unfortunately, as I am using a satellite telephone which sends and receives data at 9.6 kbps, the bmp file you sent would have taken 65 minutes to download, so I was not able to receive that. I can receive

jpg images though with ease, so if it is possible to transmit a jpg image that would be ideal.

The gif file partially got through, enough to give me a reasonable idea illustrating what you said in your email, though not perfectly. Thankfully your text file was very easy to understand. Again, if you can transmit this again in jpg format, this makes it much easier to receive. I do appreciate the effort you have gone to for this telemedicine advice.

Greatly appreciated.

Note the references to file style and size. The important thing here is the fact that even simple technology can make such a difference.

Here's another example.

I did not have time to write yesterday to thank you for your tremendous assistance, even at such a distance, after I sent you photos and clinical details last week via our telemedicine link from *****, with advice on the management of the unfortunate 22-year old man with GSW to the abdomen in Pristina University Hospital (sustained 23 June, with twelve documented perforations to small and large bowel, treated by primary repair of perfs and caecostomy).

The first two and a bit hours were spent doing a careful dissection and freeing all the small and large bowel (he had had two previous ops for his GSW) – we discovered free, small bowel contents throughout the abdomen, multiple small fistulae (at the sites of attempted repair) and collections of pus and small bowel contents, a very large fistula (actually discontinuous bowel) at the site of the disrupted caecum and previous attempted closure, and a large low jejunal fistula on the left. These findings spoke for themselves, convincing Prof ***** of the need for such exploratory surgery – and he was very happy that we were proceeding along the lines of your advice.

The semi-expected happened at 1255 hrs. ***** and I left in a hurry after handover. Dr ***** carried on and the operation was performed exactly to the guidelines of the world expert (yourself).

He proceeded to do a defunctioning proximal loop jejunostomy at the site of the first fistula, closed off the smallest fistulae, resected the larger one, and performed a right hemicolectomy. Abdo left open as laparostomy, dressed with several sheets of antibiotic impregnated tulle covered with gauze and bandage. He will supervise alternate day dressings. Dr ***** was very happy with how the operation went, and I am glad both for him and especially for the patient.

This email was a result of a digital photograph sent from 'theatre' to an advisor elsewhere.

Sir, the external fixator frame looks a little bit unstable because the connection joint is located at the centre of the fracture and one of the pins has just crossed the fraction line (it might delay healing), probably they will lose the fixation because of the great pulling strength of quadriceps muscle. They had better replace it with a more powerful one in the future. No offence just a friendly advise to my colleague.

Thanks for keeping me updated. Sincerely *****

This will let you eavesdrop on an e-exchange between some clinicians who were still in the Balkans:

I've been looking at the Balkan consults with great interest. It really is wonderful to see how the consumer computer market has made telemedicine as easy as walking down to your local CompUSA store and throwing down your credit card. I think Col ***** is justified in pointing out how it was not always so easy and how TATRC has been unjustly criticised for doing things the hard way in past years. A few years ago, the hard way was the only way. When you are first, you always have it harder and make more mistakes.

Dr ***** really points out the biggest issue with telemedicine we face today. It is no longer a technology issue. It is the willingness to take a step away from the old medical model of practitioners working in a cloistered and hierarchical structure, towards one that links us into webs. We are fortunate to live in a time where the consumer computer market is making this possible.

The e-talk continued until someone on the line came up with the following. It seems a good place to stop and a very good place to start.

I look forward to the day when all physicians and surgeons will have a hand-held computer communications-imaging device where patients can be seen, triaged, discussed, diagnosed in real time. It's not my idea. Gene Roddenberry thought it up in 1964. We are just getting damn close to having one of these things. What is the 'Post TRICORDER' profession of medicine going to look like?

In the mean time . . . God Bless our friends who are performing so bravely in the Balkans.

'If the needy were on the moon, we'd go there too.'

Mother Theresa